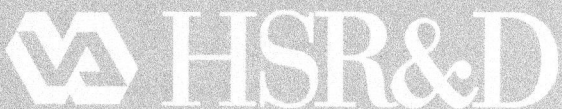

Interventions to Improve Veterans' Access to Care: A Systematic Review of the Literature

January 2011

Prepared for:
Department of Veterans Affairs
Veterans Health Administration
Health Services Research & Development Service
Washington, DC 20420

Prepared by:
Evidence-based Synthesis Program (ESP) Center
Minneapolis VA Health Care System
Minneapolis, MN
Timothy J. Wilt, MD, MPH, Director

Investigators:

Principal Investigator:
Shannon M. Kehle, PhD

Co-Investigator:
Nancy Greer, PhD

Research Associate:
Indulis Rutks, BS

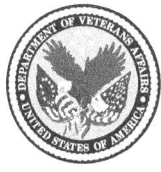

PREFACE

Health Services Research & Development Service's (HSR&D's) Evidence-based Synthesis Program (ESP) was established to provide timely and accurate syntheses of targeted healthcare topics of particular importance to Veterans Affairs (VA) managers and policymakers, as they work to improve the health and healthcare of Veterans. The ESP disseminates these reports throughout VA.

HSR&D provides funding for four ESP Centers and each Center has an active VA affiliation. The ESP Centers generate evidence syntheses on important clinical practice topics, and these reports help:

- develop clinical policies informed by evidence,
- guide the implementation of effective services to improve patient outcomes and to support VA clinical practice guidelines and performance measures, and
- set the direction for future research to address gaps in clinical knowledge.

In 2009, an ESP Coordinating Center was created to expand the capacity of HSR&D Central Office and the four ESP sites by developing and maintaining program processes. In addition, the Center established a Steering Committee comprised of HSR&D field-based investigators, VA Patient Care Services, Office of Quality and Performance, and and Veterans Integrated Service Networks (VISN) Clinical Management Officers. The Steering Committee provides program oversight and guides strategic planning, coordinates dissemination activities, and develops collaborations with VA leadership to identify new ESP topics of importance to Veterans and the VA healthcare system.

Comments on this evidence report are welcome and can be sent to Nicole Floyd, ESP Coordinating Center Program Manager, at nicole.floyd@va.gov.

Recommended citation: Kehle SM, Greer N, Rutks I, and Wilt TJ. Interventions to Improve Veterans Access to Care: A Systematic Review of the Evidence. VA-ESP Project #09-009; 2011

This report is based on research conducted by the Evidence-based Synthesis Program (ESP) Center located at the Minneapolis VA Health Care System, Minneapolis, MN funded by the Department of Veterans Affairs, Veterans Health Administration, Office of Research and Development, Health Services Research and Development. The findings and conclusions in this document are those of the author(s) who are responsible for its contents; the findings and conclusions do not necessarily represent the views of the Department of Veterans Affairs or the United States government. Therefore, no statement in this article should be construed as an official position of the Department of Veterans Affairs. No investigators have any affiliations or financial involvement (e.g., employment, consultancies, honoraria, stock ownership or options, expert testimony, grants or patents received or pending, or royalties) that conflict with material presented in the report.

TABLE OF CONTENTS

EXECUTIVE SUMMARY 1
    Background 1
    Methods 1
    Results 1
    Conclusions 2

INTRODUCTION 3

METHODS
    Topic Development 4
    Search Strategy 4
    Study Selection 5
    Data Abstraction 5
    Quality Assessment 5
    Data Synthesis 5
    Peer Review 5

RESULTS 6
    Literature Flow 6
    Key Question 1 7
    Key Question 2 12

SUMMARY AND DISCUSSION 19
    Conclusions 19
    Limitations 20
    Recommendations for Future Research 21

REFERENCES 23

FIGURES
    Figure 1. Analytic Framework 4
    Figure 2. Literature Flow Diagram for Key Questions 6

APPENDIX A. SEARCH STRATEGY 27

APPENDIX B. PEER REVIEW COMMENTS 28

APPENDIX C. EVIDENCE TABLES
    Evidence Table 1. Studies Examining Variation in Outcomes Associated with Variation in Access 31
    Evidence Table 2. Studies Examining the Efficacy of Interventions Designed to Increase Access for Veterans 40

EXECUTIVE SUMMARY

BACKGROUND

Recently, researchers within the Department of Veterans Affairs (VA) have begun to develop an updated conceptualization of access which takes into account the impact of new technology on access and places a greater focus on outcomes beyond increased access.[1] Specifically, the new conceptualization acknowledges post-access outcomes such as satisfaction, symptom levels, and functioning. As such, we sought to conduct a review of the literature that would clarify the current state of knowledge regarding the link between access to healthcare and system-level (e.g., utilization, satisfaction with care) and patient-level (quality of life, symptoms, mortality) outcomes. Given VA's continuing commitment to improving access for veterans,[2,3] we also examined the efficacy of interventions designed to improve access, with a focus on access, system-level, and patient-level outcomes (Figure 1).

The Key Questions addressed in this review are:

KEY QUESTION #1: What is the evidence that variation in veterans' ability to obtain needed health care (i.e., access) contributes to variation in system level (e.g., utilization, satisfaction) or patient level (e.g., quality of life, functional ability, mortality) outcomes?

> KEY QUESTION #1A: Does the effect of access on system and/or patient level outcomes differ by patient (e.g., demographics, overall health, illness severity), treatment (e.g., mental health, physical health), or setting (e.g., rural, urban, community, VA) characteristics?

KEY QUESTION #2: What interventions have been successful in improving access for patient populations with reduced health care access?

> KEY QUESTION #2A: Have interventions that have improved health care access led to improvements in system level and patient level outcomes?

METHODS

We searched OVID MEDLINE, CINAHL, and PsycINFO for English language articles related to access and veterans' care published in peer-reviewed journals from 1990 to June 2010. Data were abstracted from 23 articles related to Key Question #1 and 26 related to Key Question #2. We constructed evidence tables with patient characteristics, outcomes, and study quality for each study included. Due to heterogeneity in study design, patient characteristics, and outcomes, pooled analyses were not feasible.

RESULTS

KEY QUESTIONS #1 and #1a: We identified 23 studies that focused on the association between access and system-level or patient-level outcomes. Most commonly studied was the association between distance from a VA facility and utilization, primarily outpatient health and/or mental health service use. Across a variety of patient needs (e.g., treatment for substance abuse or spinal cord injury, primary care), we found fair to good evidence that increased distance from a VA facility was associated with decreased utilization. Other factors studied in relation to outpatient utilization included ability to pay for care, social support, and comorbidities. Distance, ability to pay for care, and comorbid conditions also influenced utilization of inpatient care including choice of VA or non-VA facilities. Five studies reported patient-level outcomes including two that addressed mortality. We found limited evidence that increased distance from a VA facility (one study) and longer wait time for an appointment (one study) were associated with increased mortality. We found fair evidence from six studies that identified significant interactions with the majority focused on distance and other explanatory variables such as age and diagnosis.

KEY QUESTIONS #2 and #2a: We identified 26 articles (24 unique studies) that examined the efficacy of interventions designed to increase access. Only five were randomized trials. We categorized these interventions as Community Based Outpatient Clinics, Mental Health Integration into Primary Care, Intensive Case Management, Telehealth, Outreach, CoPayments, and Other. Changes in medication copayments had the strongest evidence base with four studies. We found fair strength of evidence that increases in medication copayments decreased access / adherence to needed medications. Community Based Outpatient Clinics and Primary Care Mental Health Integration were evaluated in 6 studies each, but the studies were of low quality. There were fewer studies that evaluated other interventions (e.g., primary care mental health integration, intensive case management, telemedicine, outreach). Nineteen studies reported system-level outcomes, most often satisfaction with care and use of primary care. The majority of studies that reported satisfaction found veterans were more satisfied with care following the intervention. All but one of the studies on primary care and general medical visits found that the intervention was associated with increased utilization. Six studies reported patient-level outcomes: three found that access did not impact outcomes and one found that veterans with increased access had worse outcomes.

CONCLUSIONS

The data suggest it is possible to improve access to healthcare, although there was a lack of high quality evidence supporting the efficacy of any one intervention. There was fair evidence that increases in medication copayments decrease access / adherence to needed medications. However, future research is needed to determine if decreasing copayments increases access/ adherence. There was fair evidence of a relationship between improved access and better system-level outcomes (satisfaction and primary care utilization). There was a lack of data regarding the link between access and patient-level outcomes. Future research should focus on the quality and appropriateness of care and patient-level outcomes.

INTRODUCTION

Access to healthcare has been identified as a critical issue, both by the Department of Veterans Affairs (VA) and the larger medical community.[4-7] Access has been broadly defined as "the timely use of personal health services to achieve the best health outcomes" and has been hypothesized to have three discrete steps: 1) gaining entry into the system, 2) getting access to sites of care where patients can receive needed services, and 3) finding providers who meet the needs of the patient and with whom a productive working relationship can form.[4,6] Historically, VA has focused on the first two steps (getting access to the system and sites of care) and has adopted Demakis's[5] conceptualization of access as an individual's ability to obtain the healthcare they need within an appropriate time frame.[7]

Recently, researchers within the VA have begun to develop an updated conceptualization of access which takes into account the impact of new technology on access and places a greater focus on outcomes beyond increased access.[1] Specifically, while the definition of access remains limited to the ability to connect with needed care, the reconceptualization acknowledges post-access outcomes such as satisfaction, symptom levels, and functioning. As such, we sought to conduct a review of the literature that would clarify the current state of the knowledge regarding the link between access to healthcare (both objective and perceived access) and system-level (e.g., utilization, satisfaction with care) and patient-level (quality of life, symptoms, mortality) outcomes. Further, the VA has continued its commitment to improving access for Veterans,[2,3] and has implemented several programs designed to improve access to care for all veterans. Examples include the establishment of clinics located in areas distant from VA facilities (Community-Based Outpatient Clinics or CBOCs), mobile clinics, and increased use of telecommunications (telephone, internet, or videoconferencing). As such, we also examined the efficacy of interventions designed to improve access, with a focus on access, system-level, and patient-level outcomes (Figure 1).

The key questions addressed in this review are as follows:

KEY QUESTION #1: What is the evidence that variation in veterans' ability to obtain needed health care (i.e., access) contributes to variation in system level (e.g., utilization, satisfaction) or patient level (e.g., quality of life, functional ability, mortality) outcomes?

> KEY QUESTION #1A: Does the effect of access on system and/or patient level outcomes differ by patient (e.g., demographics, overall health, illness severity), treatment (e.g., mental health, physical health), or setting (e.g., rural, urban, community, VA) characteristics?

KEY QUESTION #2: What interventions have been successful in improving access for patient populations with reduced health care access?

> KEY QUESTION #2A: Have interventions that have improved health care access led to improvements in system level and patient level outcomes?

Figure 1. Analytic Framework

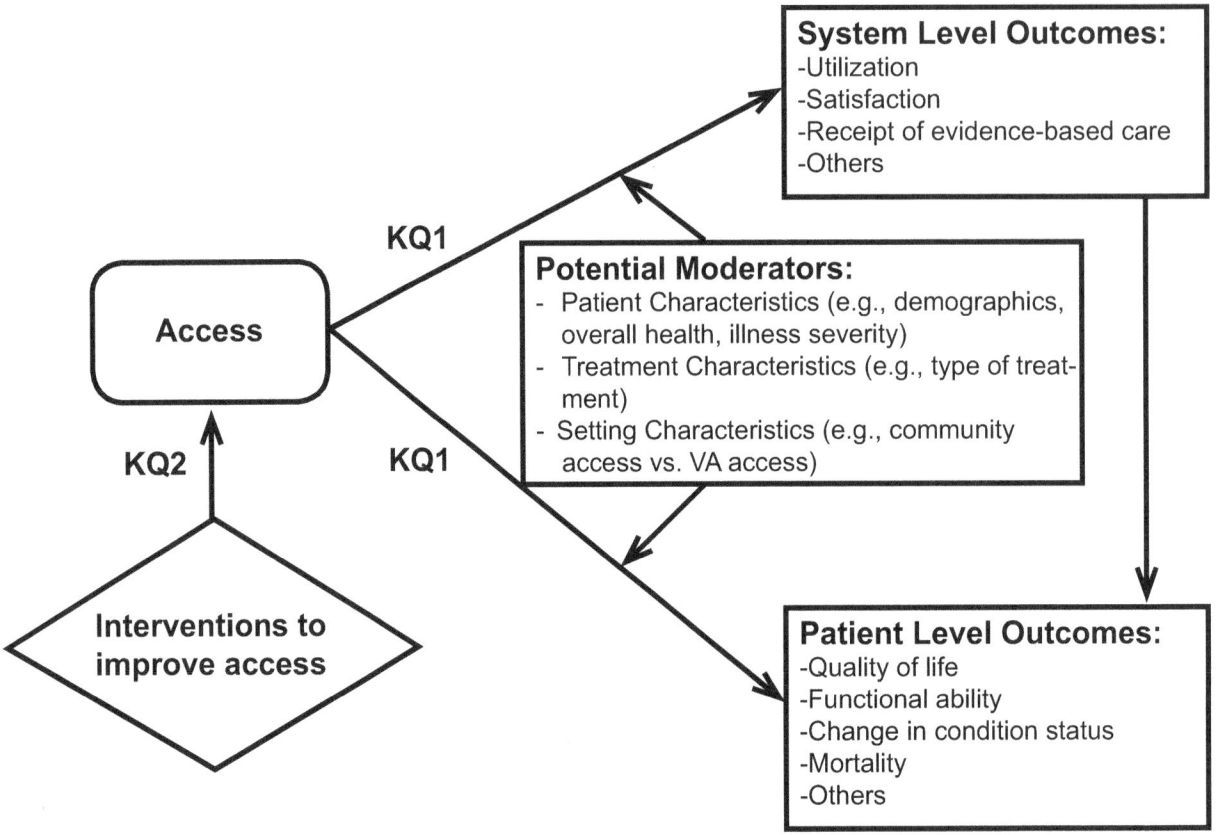

METHODS

TOPIC DEVELOPMENT, TECHNICAL EXPERT PANEL

This topic was nominated by the Planning Committee for the 2010 VA Health Services Research & Development State of the Art (SOTA) Conference on "Improving Access to VA Care" in consultation with the VA HSR&D Evidence Synthesis Program. John Fortney, PhD, Maurilio Garcia-Maldonado, MD, and Bonnie Wakefield, PhD, RN, agreed to serve on the Technical Expert Panel (TEP) for the project. The TEP members and the investigators from the Minneapolis VA Evidence-based Synthesis Program (ESP) collaborated to identify and refine the key questions.

SEARCH STRATEGY

We searched MEDLINE (OVID), CINAHL, and PsycINFO for studies published from 1990 to June, 2010. To focus the search on Veterans, we used the following MEDLINE search terms: Health Services Accessibility, access, Veterans, United States Department of Veteran Affairs, and Hospitals, Veterans (see Appendix A). Similar search terms were used in the CINAHL and PsycINFO searches. We limited the searches to articles involving human subjects ages 18 and older published in English language. All publication types were included. Additional references were identified by searching the reference lists of articles identified for inclusion.

STUDY SELECTION

Titles and abstracts identified from the search were reviewed by the investigators to identify eligible articles likely related to one or more of the key questions. Exclusion criteria were as follows:

1) Not English language
2) Not United States veteran population
3) Not published from 1990 to present
4) Not about access to health care
5) Not about outcomes of interest
6) Not peer-reviewed (including meeting abstracts and presentations).

DATA ABSTRACTION

For Key Question 1, investigators abstracted data on study design, patient characteristics, dependent and explanatory variables included in analyses, impact of access on system-level and patient-levels outcomes, and interaction terms. For Key Question 2, investigators abstracted data on study design, patient characteristics, intervention, and impact of the intervention on access, system-level, and patient-level outcomes.

QUALITY ASSESSMENT

Randomized control trials (RCTs) and cohort studies were assigned a rating of good, fair, or poor using the United States Preventive Services Task Force criteria.[8] Observational studies were rated in the domains of participant selection (e.g., appropriate recruitment of subjects/ choice of database, response rate, representativeness), outcomes assessment (e.g., valid and reliable measures, no differential or overall high loss to follow-up), and analysis (e.g., potential confounders equally distributed or adjusted for in analysis). If all three of the three criteria were rated as adequate, the study received an overall rating of fair. All other observational studies were rated as poor. For Key Question 2, all intervention types also received a strength of evidence rating (in regards to impact on access, not system- and patient-level outcomes). Interventions for which 80% or greater of the studies received a fair or good quality rating were rated as fair. All other interventions were rating as poor strength of evidence; interventions with two or fewer studies were also rated as poor.

DATA SYNTHESIS

We constructed evidence tables showing the study characteristics and results for all included studies, organized by key question and, for Key Question 2, by intervention. We compiled a summary of findings for each key question and developed conclusions based on qualitative synthesis of the findings. We did not conduct pooled analyses due to marked heterogeneity in study design, patient characteristics, and outcomes assessed.

PEER REVIEW

A draft report was reviewed by our TEP members, by participants at the 2010 "Improving Access to VA Care" State of the Art (SOTA) Conference, and by invited peer-reviewers. Reviewer comments and author responses are summarized in Appendix B.

RESULTS

LITERATURE FLOW

The OVID MEDLINE search yielded 209 references with 10 duplicates for a total of 199 unique references. The CINAHL search yielded 212 additional references and the PsycINFO search yielded 252 additional references. When the results from these searches were combined there were 663 titles and abstracts for review. From the 663 titles and abstracts, 553 references were excluded. The full text of 110 references was then reviewed and another 74 references were excluded. By hand searching reference lists from relevant articles we identified another 4 references and 9 articles were identified by a TEP member or reviewer. A total of 49 articles were included. Figure 2 details the exclusion criteria and the number of references related to each of the key questions.

Figure 2 Literature Flow Diagram (for Key Questions 1 and 2)

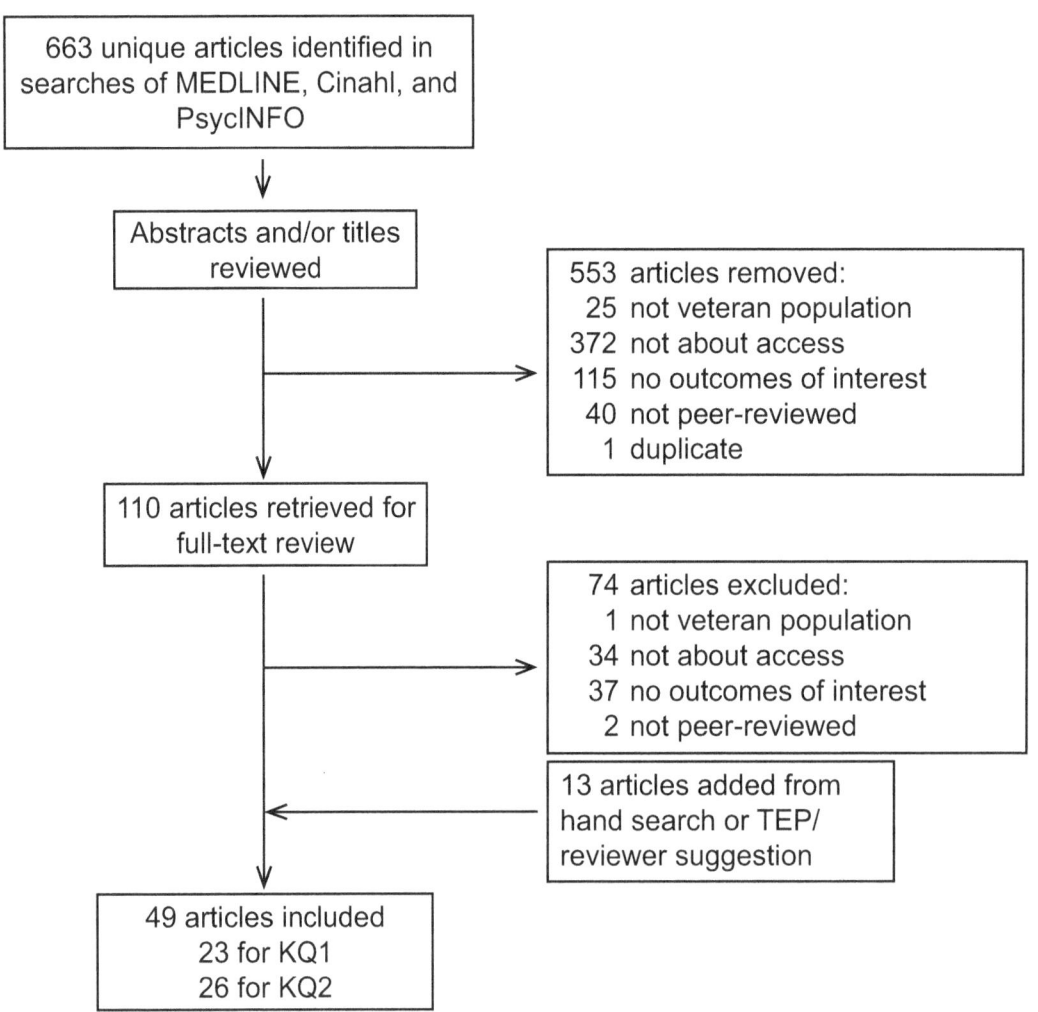

KEY QUESTION #1: WHAT IS THE EVIDENCE THAT VARIATION IN VETERANS' ABILITY TO OBTAIN NEEDED HEALTH CARE (I.E., ACCESS) CONTRIBUTES TO VARIATION IN SYSTEM-LEVEL (E.G., UTILIZATION, SATISFACTION) OR PATIENT-LEVEL (E.G., QUALITY OF LIFE, FUNCTIONAL ABILITY, MORTALITY) OUTCOMES?

We identified 23 studies representing 22 datasets that looked at the impact of access on system-level or patient-level outcomes (see Appendix C, Table 1). There were 9 cohort studies and 14 cross-sectional studies. Four studies were of good quality,[9-12] 13 were of fair quality,[13-25] and six were of poor quality.[26-31] Sample sizes in the 23 studies ranged from 109 to 3,424,699. Twenty studies enrolled veterans exclusively. In one study, 98.5% of the patients were veterans,[18] in a second study 30.5% of the participants were veterans,[31] in a third study 17% were veterans.[26] Twenty-two studies reported gender. Four of those studies included only males. In the remaining 18 studies, 93% to 98% of the participants were male. Twenty-one studies also reported age. Mean age in 11 studies that enrolled patients 18 years and older ranged from 43 to 59 years. In two studies from the same dataset that enrolled only patients 65 years and older, the mean age was 78 years. Two studies reported median age with a median of 75 years in a study that enrolled only patients age 65 and older and a median of 34 years in another study. Six studies reported number of participants in specified age intervals. Race or ethnicity data were reported in 18 studies. One study included only Native American veterans. In the remaining studies, 29% to 88% were Caucasian (reported in 13 studies), 9% to 54% were African-American (13 studies), 3% to 28% were Hispanic (4 studies), and 1% were Native American (1 study). Between 1% and 92% were reported as Other (4 studies), and 7% and 10% were Unknown (2 studies). One study reported Hispanic and non-white race/ethnicity by age and VA use categories.

Many factors can impact veterans' ability to obtain needed care. Distance to VA facilities, wait times for appointments, ability to pay for care (considering income, disability, and service connection), social support, severity of illness/comorbid conditions, and access to other care (via Medicare or private insurance) have all been investigated. In the following sections we report the evidence regarding the impact of these factors on system-level and patient-level outcomes organized by clinical service area.

SYSTEM-LEVEL OUTCOMES:

System-level outcomes, including utilization, admission, and readmission, were reported in 22 studies including 8 cohort studies and 14 cohort studies. Fifteen of the studies (14 datasets) analyzed data from national VA datasets or surveys. Three studies were of good quality, 13 were of fair quality, and 6 were of poor quality.

Outpatient services: Data from a national survey of veterans highlighted decreased use of outpatient services as distance from a VA facility increased.[13] The greatest decrease in utilization was noted for distances up to 60 miles with little change beyond. For veterans who chose to use the VA for some outpatient services, distance from the facility had a smaller additional effect on the number of visits. Increased use of VA physical and mental health services was noted for Vietnam veterans living on American Indian reservations located closer to VA facilities (in the Northern Plains region) compared to veterans living on a reservation located further from VA facilities (in the Southwest region).[29] In a nationwide study of 8,983 veterans with spinal cord injuries and disorders, use of VA outpatient services decreased as distance from a VA facility increased. Increased age, non-white race, and a history of major illness were associated with increased utilization.[20] Non-metropolitan VA patients between 18 and 44 years old were more likely (p<0.005) to report that they needed to see a doctor but could not because of cost than metropolitan VA patients or non-VA patients, or non-veterans of the same age. Among 45 to 64 year olds, VA patients, regardless of residence, were more likely to report cost as a factor than non-VA patients or non-veterans.[31]

Veterans and non-veterans with human immunodeficiency virus (HIV) reported problems with transportation time (greater than 1 hour [17%] or greater than 30 minutes [55%]) and location (34%). In addition to travel barriers, patients with HIV also reported problems with office hours (48%), wait time for urgent appointments (greater than 2 days [23%] or greater than 1 day [50%]), office wait time (greater than 2 hours [32%] or greater than 1 hour [54%], and cost of care (49%).[26]

Homeless veterans in 9 states who had serious mental illness were more likely to use VA services if they resided in cities with VA medical centers or hospitals, if they had service-connected disabilities, or if they received non-service connected VA pensions.[27] A regional study that enrolled homeless veterans found increased use of VA services among those living in metropolitan areas and among those receiving financial support though the Department of Veterans Affairs.[28]

Patients who were discharged following treatment for acute myocardial infarction (MI) were less likely to receive outpatient care within 30 days or within 90 days if they lived more than 20 miles from the admitting hospital. The analysis was based on data from over 4,000 veterans nationwide. Other factors associated with increased likelihood of receiving outpatient care within 30 days were service connected disability, age over 55 years, comorbid conditions, discharge from a teaching hospital, and revascularization procedure while a history of alcohol abuse was associated with decreased likelihood. A similar pattern was seen for the likelihood of one or more visits within 90 days except that alcoholism, type of hospital, and comorbidity were not related.[10]

Three large studies (2 that used data from national datasets, 1 that used data from 33 VA treatment programs) evaluated use of VA care following inpatient treatment for alcoholism, psychiatry, and / or substance abuse.[9,14,25] Patients who lived closer to VA facilities were more likely to attend an aftercare appointment[9,25] and were more likely to use outpatient medical services.[14] Urban residing (with distance held constant) and unmarried patients were less likely to attend aftercare for alcohol dependence.[9] Patients receiving VA compensation payments, those with a psychiatric diagnosis (as opposed to substance abuse), and those who had mental health follow-up within 30 days of discharge were also more likely to have received outpatient medical services following an inpatient stay for psychiatry or substance abuse.[14] Older age, married status, service-connected eligibility, psychiatric comorbidity, substance use disorder, and being a patient at a teaching hospital were associated with increased likelihood of receiving aftercare following inpatient substance abuse care; medical comorbidities were associated with decreased likelihood.[25]

Three studies presented data on patients receiving mental health care. In a study that enrolled veterans receiving mental health services at 2 VA mental health centers, increased outpatient use of mental health services was associated with fewer reported access problems and no social support although the greatest predictor of use was clinical need.[16] Among patients (nationwide) with bipolar disorder, schizophrenia, or other psychoses, the number of psychiatric and non-psychiatric outpatient visit days decreased as distance from the VA outpatient service increased. Patients who had initial contact at a non-psychiatric clinic, a higher comorbidity rating, or resided in a rural area had fewer outpatient psychiatric visit days while those who were older, married, female, rural, had an initial visit at a non-psychiatric facility, or had a higher comorbidity rating had more outpatient non-psychiatric visit days.[21] In a similar population, an increased risk of a 12 month gap in VA health system utilization was associated with residence a greater distance from a VA facility, homelessness, and a recent inpatient stay while a decreased risk of a 12 month gap was associated with residence in a county with greater availability of VA inpatient beds, older age, female gender, married status, VA service connection, higher comorbidity score, and a diagnosis of schizophrenia. An increased risk of a 12 month gap in mental health services was associated with residence a greater distance from VA psychiatric services, increased age, female gender, homelessness, higher comorbidity score, and recent inpatient stay. A decreased risk of a gap in mental health services was associated with married status, VA service connection, and a diagnosis of schizophrenia.[22]

Use of VA or non-VA health and mental health services was the focus of three additional studies. In one study, with data from over 1.4 million outpatients, there was an increase in the exclusive use of a VA facility as distance from the facility decreased. There was also greater exclusive use of outpatient VA facilities among patients with a higher VA priority designation and those living in counties with a higher level of poverty. Urban residents and those living in counties with a higher number of hospital beds were less likely to rely exclusively on VA care.[19] A second study, with over 20,000 survey respondents, reported increased use of VA outpatient health and mental health services among those younger, unmarried, unemployed, and lacking health insurance. Greater use of VA health services (but not mental health services) was also associated with VA disability rating and poorer physical health. Non-VA health visits were associated with older age, female gender, college education, unemployment, disability rating and poorer physical and mental health. Non-VA mental health visits were associated with younger age, female gender, college education, unmarried status, unemployment, urban residence, and poorer physical and mental health.[15] The third study, with data from over 1.9 million veterans, reported increased reliance on VA care (outpatient and overall) if the differential distance (distance from residence to VA facilities and non-VA facilities) was lower. There was also greater reliance on VA care by veterans with disability or low income priority classifications and those with mental health or substance abuse conditions.[24]

Inpatient services: One study focused on facility wait time for care and admission for an ambulatory care sensitive condition (ACSC) such as asthma, diabetes, or chronic obstructive pulmonary disease. Hospitalization for an ACSC would likely be avoided if the patient were to receive appropriate outpatient care in a timely manner. The analysis included data from 33,431 veterans age 65 and older who visited a geriatric outpatient clinic. The probability of admission for an ACSC was significantly greater ($p<0.05$) for veterans who visited facilities with wait times of 29 days or more compared to visits to facilities with wait times of less than 22.5 days. Age, previous ACSC hospitalization, higher comorbidity index, and diagnosis of cancer or endocrine, heart, or pulmonary disease were also associated with increased risk of hospitalization.[12]

Patients who presented for emergency psychiatric care at one VA facility were more likely to be admitted for treatment if they lived more than 60 miles from the facility. Age greater than 65 years and lower score on the Global Assessment of Functioning (GAF) were also associated with increased likelihood of admission.[17] A study based at 2 VA mental health centers found that increased inpatient hospitalization for mental health services was associated with homelessness although the greatest predictor was clinical need.[16]

Veterans with spinal cord injuries and disorders had lower inpatient utilization if they lived a greater distance from the facility while history of major illness was associated with increased inpatient utilization.[20]

The impact of access to care on readmission was reported in two studies. Increased distance, expressed as "close," "medium," or "far," from the county where the VA admitting facility was located, was associated with a non-significant, incremental, 18% increase in the risk of early (within 30 days) readmission. The veterans enrolled in this study were discharged from the internal medicine, surgery, intermediate care, or neurology services. The probability of readmission was also increased if the patient had two or more surgeries or their readmission risk was rated above "very low."[18] Using national VA databases, distance to care was not associated with an increased risk of readmission following treatment for MI. Age greater than 65 years, comorbid conditions, and receipt of any VA ambulatory care within 90 days were associated with increased risk of readmission.[10]

Three studies explored choice of VA or non-VA inpatient services. An analysis of data from over 400,000 veterans with inpatient admissions yielded results similar to those observed for outpatient utilization notably decreased exclusive use of VA services as distance to the VA increased. Age, urban residence, VA priority level, and poverty level were also factors associated with choice of inpatient services.[19] A study of over 2 million hospital admissions for any of 14 high-risk elective surgeries among veterans 65 years or older found that 89% of heart surgeries, 85% of vascular surgeries, and 79% of cancer resections were performed in non-VA hospitals with little difference based on place of residence. The study also differentiated high performing from low performing hospitals and reported that, regarding travel time to high performing hospitals, urban residents had the least travel burden.[31] Data from over 1.9 million veterans suggested that patients with transplant and amputation aggregated condition categories (ACCs) were more likely to rely on the VA for inpatient care. Other ACCs associated with inpatient VA care included infectious and parasitic disorders, substance abuse, mental health disorders, and eye disorders.[24]

Pharmacy utilization: One study evaluated use of VA pharmacy services. The nationwide study included veterans enrolled in both VA and Medicare programs. Enrollment in a Medicare plan with pharmacy benefits, age over 65 years, income of $20,000 or greater, female gender, VA priority status requiring copayment for medications, Medicare state buy-in, resident of a metropolitan statistical area, and being a patient at a teaching hospital were associated with decreased likelihood of using a VA pharmacy. Veterans of Hispanic race and of poorer health status were more likely to use the VA pharmacy.[23]

PATIENT-LEVEL OUTCOMES:

In contrast to system-level outcomes, patient-level outcomes, including mortality, perceived health, and quality of life, were only reported in 5 studies. Three were cohort studies (two of good quality, one of fair quality) and 2 were cross-sectional studies (both of fair quality).

Two nationwide studies evaluated mortality.[10,11] Patients discharged following hospitalization for MI and living more than 20 miles away from the admitting hospital had a significantly higher risk of dying within 1 year compared to individuals living within 20 miles. Age greater than 55 years and presence of comorbid conditions were also associated with increased risk of mortality while undergoing revascularization or receiving VA ambulatory care within 90 days after the index visit was associated with decreased risk of death.[10] Based on the dataset of veterans 65 years of age and older who were seen for outpatient geriatric services at VA medical centers (Prentice, 2008), patients who visited facilities with wait times of 31 days or longer had a higher risk of death within 6 months than those who visited facilities with wait times of less than 31 days. Other factors significantly associated with increased risk of mortality included increased age, 50% or greater service connected disability, preventable hospitalization, higher comorbidity index, or diagnosis of cancer or endocrine, neurological, psychiatric, pulmonary, or "other" disease. Female gender was associated with decreased risk of mortality.[11]

Two smaller studies examined the impact of access on either quality of life in individuals with human immunodeficiency virus (HIV) or mental health among patients receiving mental health services. In 205 veteran and non-veteran patients with HIV, better overall health related quality of life (HRQOL) was associated with better perceived access to care ($p<0.01$). Included in the perceived access measure were affordability, availability, and convenience of care along with accessibility of specialists. The relationship between HRQOL and temporal access (transportation and waiting times) was not significant[26]. In another study, treatment access was not associated with mental health outcomes (Global Assessment of Function or Behavior and Symptom Identification Scale-24) among 421 patients receiving mental health services at 2 VA sites.[16]

Self-reported health and days of poor health in the preceding 30 days were reported in one study of over 45,000 veterans and non-veterans. The poorest health was reported by veterans currently in VA care, in particular, non-metropolitan residents age 45 and older. Veterans in VA care, regardless of residence, reported a higher number of days of poor health (physical, mental, or limiting activities) in the past 30 days when compared to veterans not in VA care or non-veterans.[30]

KEY QUESTION #1A: DOES THE EFFECT OF ACCESS ON SYSTEM AND/OR PATIENT LEVEL OUTCOMES DIFFER BY PATIENT, TREATMENT, OR SETTING CHARACTERISTICS?

Six studies evaluated the effect of interactions on system level factors.[9,13,21,24,26,28] All but one of the studies[26] included either a national sample of veterans[13,21,24,28] or veterans treated at multiple sites.[9] There were two cohort studies (one of good quality and one of fair quality) and four cross-sectional studies (two of fair quality and two of poor quality).

The effect of distance on the number of outpatient visits, both psychiatric[21] and non-psychiatric[13,21], as well as reliance on VA care[24] was greater for older patients. Patients with a

11

diagnosis of schizophrenia were also more affected by distance than those with bipolar disorder.[21] Among patients scheduled to attend an aftercare appointment within 30 days following an inpatient alcohol dependency program, older patients and those with a rural residence were more negatively impacted by distance.[9] On a scale of 0 (worst possible access) to 100 (best possible access), the access scores for transportation time to appointment were lower for patients infected with HIV and who had VA insurance compared to those who had California Medicaid insurance (p<0.05). The access scores for covering cost of care and availability of hospital care were higher for VA patients than for uninsured (non-VA) patients while the scores for office wait time and availability of emergency care were higher for VA patients than for uninsured or California Medicaid patients (all p<0.05).[26] Among homeless veterans, the effect of metropolitan/non-metropolitan status on use of VA facilities varied based on age, military service era, monthly income, time homeless, and past alcohol or drug dependency.[28]

KEY QUESTIONS #2 AND #2A: WHAT INTERVENTIONS HAVE BEEN SUCCESSFUL IN IMPROVING ACCESS FOR PATIENT POPULATIONS WITH REDUCED HEALTH CARE ACCESS? HAVE INTERVENTIONS THAT HAVE IMPROVED HEALTH CARE ACCESS LED TO IMPROVEMENTS IN SYSTEM LEVEL AND PATIENT LEVEL OUTCOMES?

We identified 26 articles (24 unique studies) that assessed interventions designed to improve veterans' access to healthcare (see Appendix C, Table 2). We only included articles that provided data regarding the intervention's impact on actual access (observable, measurable dimensions), perceived access (self-reported, subjective dimensions), or satisfaction with access.[1] During abstraction, we found that the articles reported on six distinct types of interventions. The results are grouped by those interventions.

COMMUNITY BASED OUTPATIENT CLINICS (CBOCs):

Detailed Description

In order to increase access to primary care for veterans living in rural or other underserved geographical areas, the VA began opening satellite primary care clinics, known as CBOCs. Four of the articles[32-35] utilized quasi-experimental designs to examine the impact of the opening of CBOCs on access factors. All four studies found that the opening of CBOCs had a positive impact on geographic accessibility as evidenced by the CBOCs attracting more users new to the VA than VA Medical Centers (VAMCS), a decrease in travel distance to the closest VA facility for those in CBOC catchment areas, and higher rates of accessing VA medical services in counties with a CBOC. A number of system-level outcomes were also identified. It was found that CBOC patients had more primary care visits and that decreases in travel distance significantly predicted increases in the number of primary care encounters.

Findings regarding the utilization of specialty care were mixed. Fortney et al.[32] found that CBOC patients had fewer specialty care encounters, while Fortney et al.[33,34] found that those in CBOC catchment areas had more ancillary and extended care physical health visits. Finally, in counties with CBOCs that offered specialty mental health services, more veterans accessed mental health services. Importantly, CBOCs did not have a significant impact on a number of access and system-level outcomes (e.g., days between discharge and outpatient follow-up, hospital admissions, inpatient days) and the impact on some system-level outcomes were small and may not be clinically significantly. For example, Fortney et al.[33] reported that those in the CBOC catchment area only had 0.5 more primary care visits in the 18-months post-implementation than pre-implementation. None of the studies provided data on patient-level outcomes.

It is important to note that while these studies found that CBOCs had a positive impact on geographical access, a vast majority of veterans residing in catchment areas (approximately 85%) still did not receive VA care.[35] However, data suggest that high priority groups (those with service-connection or chronic diseases) may be experiencing greater benefits from the opening of CBOCs. For example, veterans in CBOC catchment areas with alcohol-related and hypertension diagnoses attended more primary care visits, while those with diabetes attended more mental health and ancillary services than veterans not in a CBOC catchment area[33]. Further, Rosenheck et al.[35] found that veterans who were service-connected for any disorder (7.6% increase for those with no new CBOCs; 9.6% increase for those with new CBOCs) and those who were service-connected for non-mental health problems (7.3% increase for those with no new CBOCs; 9.4% increase for those with new CBOCs) had a significant increase in VA services. Finally, three studies found that CBOC veterans differ from VAMC veterans on demographic factors; those at CBOCS were found to be older, more often male, more often Caucasian, less often African American or Hispanic, more often married, and less often service connected than veterans seen at the parent VAMCs.

Two studies examined veterans' satisfaction with access and other aspects of care at CBOCs. Borowsky et al.[36] reported that veterans using CBOCs reported better access / timeliness and were more likely to report waits of less than 20 minutes than veterans getting care at VAMCs. Further, veterans using CBOCs more often reported having good or excellent visits and reported fewer problems with their visits. Morgester et al.[37] examined differences in veterans who received care from a CBOC, those who lived in a CBOC catchment area who did not use VA care, and those who received care from a VAMC. All three groups reported few access problems; they had few problems finding the clinic, found the hours of operation convenient, and were satisfied with care. Although no statistical comparisons were conducted, differences between the three groups were small. No patient-level outcomes were reported for either study.

Summary of findings

We identified six studies that examined the impact of the opening or use of CBOCs on veterans' access to health care. None of the studies were randomized trials, although four utilized quasi-experimental designs in which cohorts were compared both pre- and post-implementation. Overall, the sample sizes were large, with one being VA-wide. Four of the studies were of fair quality, while 2 were poor quality. The overall strength of the evidence was poor.

All six studies found that CBOCs had a positive impact on various measures of access; four studies found an association between the opening of CBOCs and objective measures of access to primary care while two studies found that veterans were satisfied with CBOCs' accessibility. Five of the studies reported system-level outcomes. Overall, increased access was associated with increased primary care use, while findings regarding specialty care were mixed. No studies reported patient-level outcomes.

PRIMARY CARE MENTAL HEALTH INTEGRATION:

Detailed Description

Two articles examined the impact of integrating mental health services into a primary care clinic, with the specific goal of improving access and outcomes for veterans with depression.[38,39] Watts et al.[39] conducted a quasi-experimental study examining a primary care clinic before and after the PCMH integration at a VAMC and associated CBOCs. The mental health services involved co-location of mental health services in the primary care clinic, collaborations between the primary care and mental health staff, advance or open access to mental health providers within the primary care clinic, and the use of standardized instruments for the assessment of mental health conditions. After PCMH integration, they found that more veterans at the VAMC received care for depression and fewer veterans received no depression treatment. Further they found that more veterans received care in mental health clinics and wait times for an appointment in the mental health clinics decreased substantially. None of these differences were significant at the CBOCs. In regard to systems outcomes, more veterans at the VAMC received "optimal depression treatment" following integration. No patient-level variables were reported. Shiner et al.[38] reported on the effect of implementing five differing models of PCMH integration at one VAMC and four CBOCs. At the VAMC, the PCMH integration model was the same as described above. CBOC-A offered walk-in access one day per week, assessment by both a psychotherapy and psychopharmacologically oriented provider, and standardized assessments. CBOC-B had a psychotherapist on the primary care team and had back-up telepsychiatry services by appointment. CBOC-C did not have PCMH integration, but had a mental health clinic on-site. CBOC-D did not offer mental health services. Following implementation, the VAMC and CBOC-A had nearly identical results, with both experiencing increases in the number of veterans receiving mental health care in four days and 30 days, and the number of veterans receiving optimal care. The less intensive CBOC-B also had an increase in the number of veterans receiving care within 30 days and the number of veterans receiving optimal care. There were no differences for CBOC-C or CBOC-D. No system- or patient-level outcomes were assessed.

Two articles examined implementing primary care clinics into existing mental health / substance use clinics.[40,41] Druss et al.[40] conducted a randomized trial to examine the efficacy of implementing a primary care in the mental health clinic. In regard to access, veterans randomized to PCMH integration reported significantly better satisfaction with access to care. The two conditions also yielded significant differences on a number of systems-level variables; those in PCMH integration had more primary care visits, fewer ER visits, received more preventive services, and reported greater satisfaction across a number of domains. Finally, in regard to patient-level outcomes, veterans assigned to PCMH integration had better physical component SF-36 scores at one-year post randomization; there was no difference on the mental component score. Saxon et al.[41] conducted a similar study in which they randomized veterans receiving care in a substance use clinic to receive primary care from a clinic located within the substance use clinic or through a medical clinic (treatment as usual). The integrated condition fared better on measures of access, including length of wait for initial primary care visit, odds of attending a rescheduled initial visit, and the likelihood of attending at least one primary care visit. However, there was no difference on the likelihood of attending the initially scheduled appointment. In regard to system-level outcomes, those assigned to PCMH integration condition were more likely to attend return primary care visits and had more primary care visits during the study period, were less likely to seek non-VA care, and were more likely to remain engaged in substance use treatment at 60 days (although not at 6 or 12 months). Mean days in substance use treatment did not differ. There were no sustained differences in ER visits or hospital admissions. There were no group differences on patient-level outcomes, including the SF-36 (both physical and mental composite scores) or substance use disorder outcomes.

Finally, one study reported on the effort to integrate primary care, mental health, and services for homeless veterans.[42,43] The quasi-experimental design compared homeless veterans with substance use problems and serious mental illness both before and after the opening of the integrated clinic. Within the integrated clinic, veterans were evaluated in a screening clinic and quickly referred to other services, all of which were housed within the same building. The goal was to have the primary care appointment occur on the day of screening. The intervention did result in shorter wait times for an initial primary care appointment; the PHMC integration group had, on average, less than a day lapse, while the usual care group waited approximately 2 months for their initial visit. In regards to system-level outcomes, the PCMH group received more preventive services, had a higher number of primary care visits, and had lower levels of ER use. There were no differences in rates of admission, inpatient days, or the number of veterans receiving primary care. There were no significant differences in the patient-level variable of physical health status.

Summary of Findings

We identified six articles (five unique studies) that examined the impact of primary care mental health (PCMH) integration on veterans' access to health care services. Two studies examined the integration of primary care into mental health clinics; two examined the integration of mental health into primary care clinics; and one study (two articles) examined the integration of mental health, primary care, and homeless services. Two of the studies were randomized trials, the others were quasi-experimental. The overall strength of the evidence was poor; one study was of high quality, two of fair quality, and three were low quality.

All five found that integration led to improvements in objective or self-reported access. Two studies specifically examined access to optimal treatments and found that PCMH led to more veterans receiving optimal depression care. Three studies found associations between increased access and more primary care visits. Three studies reported on patient-level outcomes; results were mixed.

INTENSIVE CASE MANAGEMENT:

Two studies (one good, one poor quality) examined the effect of intensive case management on access.[44,45] The overall strength of the evidence was poor. Both intensive case management programs had a number of goals, including increasing access to needed services for veterans already within the VA system who had high levels of health care needs. Ritchie et al.[44] examined the impact of the Coordination and Advocacy for Rural Elders (CARE) program, which was designed to improve the health and functioning and to extend the length of independent living for elderly rural veterans. This is done, in part, through increasing access to health services. Veterans in the care program received multiple, standardized assessments through which a provider identified problems, developed a care plan, and tracked the resolution of problems. In regard to access, it was found that over 56% of veteran received a medical referral or linkage following the assessments. No system- or patient-level outcomes were assessed.

Weinberger et al.[45] conducted a randomized trial in which hospitalized veterans with diabetes, chronic obstructive pulmonary disease, or congestive heart failure, who did not have ongoing primary care, were assigned to either treatment as usual or an intensive primary care program. The primary care program was designed to increase access to primary care through both inpatient and outpatient components. While the veteran was still in the hospital, a primary care doctor and nurse each made visits to assess current functioning and post-discharge needs, and the primary care nurse made an appointment for the veteran to visit the primary care clinic within one week of discharge. Following discharge, the nurse called the veteran within two days to assess any problems and to remind the veteran of his upcoming appointment. Appointment reminders were sent and missed-visit protocols were implemented as needed. During the first primary care appointment, both the nurse and doctor reviewed and updated the treatment plan. In regard to access, the data showed that the median time from hospital discharge to primary care was shorter and self-reported satisfaction with access was higher for the intervention group. The two groups differed on system-level outcomes, with intervention veterans being more satisfied with care, more likely to visit a general medicine clinic, and less likely to visit specialty care. Surprisingly, those in the intervention condition were more likely to be readmitted to the hospital, readmitted sooner, and have more days of rehospitalization. There were no differences on patient-level outcomes (SF-36).

TELEMEDICINE:

Detailed Descriptions

Two studies (a cohort study and a RCT) examined the efficacy of using telemedicine as a method for patients to communicate with existing providers.[46,47] Barnett et al.[46] examined the use of telehealth messaging in older, at-risk, veterans with type two diabetes, while Hopp et al.[47] conducted a randomized trial to determine the impact of telehealth messaging on veterans receiving home care services. Both telehealth programs involved the veteran updating the nurse on current symptoms and problems via the telehealth device, which transmitted both video and sound. In the Hopp et al.[47] study, some units also had monitoring devices (e.g., blood pressure cuffs), which would directly transmit data to the nurse. During the telehealth sessions, the nurse could have discussed concerns with the veteran, provided disease management suggestions, made referrals as appropriate, and reminded the veteran to continue with his treatment plan (e.g., take medication, exercise). The telehealth programs appeared to have a positive impact on access; Hopp et al.[47] reported that contacts with VA providers increased and Barnett et al.[46] found that care-coordinator initiated primary care visits increased by 8.9% following the implementation of telehealth. However, the findings regarding outcomes were less promising. Hopp et al.[47] did not find any group differences in system-level outcomes (e.g., satisfaction, utilization variables); neither did Barnett et al.[46] after controlling for baseline A1c levels. Hopp et al.[47] did find that the intervention group had better scores on the mental component summary of the Health Related Quality of Life Scale as compared to the treatment as usual group; no other patient-level variables were significant (e.g., physical component score).

The other two telemedicine studies examined the utility of telemedicine in receiving specialty care consultations from off-site providers. Wakefield et al.[48] examined the use of telehealth to receive a variety of specialty consultations from specialists at a VAMC for veterans in a long term care facility, while Wilkins et al.[49] evaluated the feasibility of using telehealth to receive consultation from a multidisciplinary wound care team for veterans at a VAMC without such a team. In both studies, the veterans reported that telemedicine was easier and more convenient than travelling to meet with a specialist and a large majority of veterans were satisfied with telemedicine. No system- or patient-level outcomes were assessed.

Summary of Findings

We identified four studies that examined the use of telemedicine. Two studies were of fair quality and two were of poor quality, leading to an overall rating of poor. Two studies examined the efficacy of using telemedicine as a method for patients to communicate with existing providers,[46,47] while two studies examined the use of telemedicine to consult with off-site specialists.[48,49] One of the studies was an RCT of fair quality, the other three were non-experimental designs. Two studies found that veterans found telemedicine to be as, or more, convenient than in person appointments and two found that the use of telemedicine was associated with increased access / referrals to providers. One study[47] (the RCT) examined patient-level outcomes; the intervention had a positive impact on the mental component of the health-related quality of life scale.

OUTREACH:

One fair-quality RCT examined the impact of outreach efforts on veterans' access to health care. McFall et al.[50] conducted a randomized trial in which Vietnam veterans who were service-connected for posttraumatic stress disorder (PTSD) were either randomized to the outreach intervention or to a no-intervention control. Those in the intervention condition received a mailing which included information regarding PTSD treatment services and contained a letter from the director of the PTSD program inviting them to seek care and providing them with three options for responding (return a postcard, call the study coordinator, or come to the walk-in clinic). The second component of the intervention was a direct phone call to the veteran by the study coordinator. The primary purpose of the call was to inquire about barriers to seeking care, but the study authors deemed it as part of the intervention because during the phone call, veterans could ask about services, discuss and address barriers to care, or schedule an appointment. The outreach did have a positive impact on access; more veterans in the outreach condition scheduled (19% vs. 7% of the intent-to-treat sample) and presented (approximately 15% vs. 7%) for an intake session. In addition, they were more likely to attend at least one follow-up session. No patient-level outcomes were assessed.

COPAYMENTS:

Detailed Descriptions

While the VA is generally considered an open-access healthcare system in which cost does not present a significant barrier, an increase in medication copayment rates from $2 to $7 provided a unique opportunity to examine the impact of copayments on access to needed medications within the VA. We identified four cohort studies that examined the impact of the copayment increase on (a) veterans with prescriptions for diabetic, hypertensive, or hyperlipidemic medications,[51] (b) veterans with a diagnosis of schizophrenia or schizoaffective disorder,[52] (c) veterans on lipid-lowering medications[53], and (d) a random sample of VA pharmacy users.[54] Maciejewski et al.[51] found that while adherence was similar between veterans with and without a copayment prior to the cost increase, afterward, veterans with a copayment were significantly less adherent than veterans without a copayment (60% vs. 69% for those with diabetes and 76% vs. 80% for those with hypertension at the end of the study). Similarly, among veterans using lipid-lowering medications, while lipid-medication use decreased overall during the course of the study, the decrease was more pronounced in those with a copayment[53]. Zeber et al.[52] found that copayments had a negative impact on adherence. For total prescriptions (medical and psychiatric) and medical prescriptions, while both the copayment exempt and non-exempt groups increased their use of medications over the study period, the non-exempt group did so at a significantly slower rate. For psychiatric medications, those exempt from copayments increased their use throughout the study period, while those with a copayment decreased their use nearly 25% following the price increase. Further, veterans with a copayment were 5% more likely to have a psychiatric admission following the price increase. Finally, Stroupe et al.[54] found that among a random sample of VA pharmacy users, those with a copayment received 8% fewer 30-day refills than those without payments.

Summary of Findings

We identified four studies that examined the impact of the copayment increase on veterans' adherence to medications. All four studies were of fair quality and the overall strength of evidence was fair. All of the studies found that increases in medication copayments led to decreases in medication adherence. One study[52] examined system-level outcomes and found that following the price increase, veterans with a copayment had a greater increase in the rate of psychiatric hospitalization than copayment exempt veterans. No studies reported patient-level outcomes.

OTHER ACCESS INTERVENTIONS:

We identified three additional studies that examined the effect of intervention on access. All three studies were of poor study quality. Two of those examined access to specific medical services: treatment for hepatitis[55] and specialty rehabilitation care following a lower-extremity amputation.[56] Hagedorn et al.[55] implemented a Healthy Liver Program (the goal of which was to increase access to the prevention, identification, and treatment of hepatitis) into a substance abuse clinic. The intervention included testing for all veterans at the time of intake, scheduling veterans who were entering the clinic into an educational healthy liver group, administration of vaccinations, and referrals to the hepatitis clinic as necessary. Following the intervention, testing for hepatitis increased significantly and 94% of appropriate veterans started a vaccine series. Approximately 86% of veterans complied with a 1-month booster requirement and 60% complied with the 6-month booster. In regard to system-level outcomes, 78% of those who learned they had hepatitis attended their intake at the hepatitis clinic.

Bates et al.[56] examined differences in rates of referral and outcomes for veterans with a lower-extremity amputation who were at VAMCs with and without Specialized Rehabilitation Units (SRUs). The SRUs are multidisciplinary specialty teams which were hypothesized to increase awareness toward rehabilitation, which would increase access to helpful rehabilitation services. Contrary to expectations, Bates et al.[56] found that the presence of a SRU did not increase the likelihood that a veteran would be referred for rehabilitation services, however, those within a SRU VAMC were more likely to receive specialty, rather than general rehabilitation.

Finally, Rodriguez et al.[57] conducted a qualitative study to examine elderly African American veterans' reaction to a mobile geriatric care unit (MGU). The MGU was a vehicle with a check-in area, bathroom, patient education room, and examination room equipped to perform standard preventive care. The qualitative analyses revealed that veterans commented on the accessibility of care 26 times in 18 interviews. The comments were related to geographic proximity, hours of operation, and wait time. In regard to system-level outcomes, veterans mentioned quality of care 28 times. No patient-level outcomes were assessed.

SUMMARY AND DISCUSSION

CONCLUSIONS

Key Questions #1 and #1a: For outpatient care, the majority of studies we identified focused on the association between distance from a VA facility and utilization of VA services for either physical or mental health needs. Increased distance from a VA facility was consistently associated with decreased utilization (fair to good evidence). The pattern was observed for veterans in need of primary care services as well as follow-up care for substance abuse, mental illness, HIV, or spinal cord injury. Another important factor in utilization of VA services was ability to pay for care. Many studies reported increased VA care and use of VA care rather than non-VA care by veterans who were homeless, had an income- or disability-related priority status, or who were service connected. Social support and the presence of comorbid conditions were also factors although the results were less consistent.

For inpatient care, higher admission and readmission rates were generally associated with increased distance from the admitting facility and with increased comorbidity scores. The choice to utilize VA or non-VA inpatient care was inversely related to distance in one study. The condition for which inpatient care was needed was also a factor. One study of facility wait times found increased probability of admission for an ambulatory care sensitive condition for patients visiting facilities with wait times of 29 days or longer.

Few studies included patient-level outcomes. There is limited information about the association between access to care and mortality, quality of life, and perceived health.

Key Questions #2 and #2a: Taken as a whole, the results suggest that access to healthcare can be improved through structural / organizational interventions. All of the articles reported an association between the intervention and at least one measure of access (actual, perceived, or satisfaction with access). The evidence was strongest (fair support) for interventions regarding medication copayments. All four studies included in the review found that increasing medication copayments negatively impacted adherence. Further, the one study that examined system-level outcomes found that the copayment increase led to increased levels of psychiatric hospitalization. However, it is important to note that it is unclear whether decreasing copayments would improve adherence / increase access.

The implementation of CBOCs and PCMH are also promising strategies that warrant more rigorous examination, as the existing studies were generally of low quality. Four studies found a positive association between the opening of CBOCs and access to primary care, while two studies found that veterans were satisfied with CBOCs' accessibility. While none of the CBOC articles were randomized trials, four were fair quality, cohort designs and the sample sizes for a majority of the studies were large, with one being VA-wide. There were six studies that presented data regarding the impact of PCMH integration on access. Two articles examined the impact of integrating mental health services into primary care clinics. Both found that PCMH integration increased access to mental health services. Further, it was found that less intensive models of PCMH implemented within CBOCs also had a significant positive impact on access. Two of the articles, both randomized trials (one fair quality, one good quality), evaluated the efficacy of implementing primary care into mental health clinics. The integration led to self-reported and objective increases in access. Finally, one study (two articles), found that integrating homeless, mental health, and primary care services reduced wait times to primary care to less than one day. Thus, PCMH integration show promise, however, more research on each of the models of integration is needed.

The other intervention that showed promise but requires additional research, was the use of telemedicine. Four studies, one of which was a fair quality RCT, showed that veterans found telemedicine convenient and it led to increased access to providers. The ability of telemedicine to improve access deserves further study, especially in light of findings that interventions delivered via telemedicine yield equivalent outcomes to in-person treatment (e.g., Tuerk et al.[58]).

A number of other interventions (intensive case management, outreach strategies, copayments, mobile access units, and availability / integration of specialty care) each had one to two articles which examined their efficacy. While all of the interventions either resulted in referrals to additional care, improved wait times, better access to needed treatments (medication), or self-reported satisfaction with access, all require further validation.

Nineteen of the 24 unique studies reported system-level outcomes. The two most frequently reported system-level outcomes were satisfaction with care and number of primary care visits. A large majority of studies that reported satisfaction found that veterans were more satisfied with care following the intervention; the remaining studies found no difference in satisfaction. In regard to primary care and general medical visits, all but one of the studies that reported on those outcomes found that the intervention was associated with increased utilization. Findings regarding the use of specialty care and hospitalization were mixed. Although few studies reported on the outcomes, results were consistent regarding an increase in preventive care and improved engagement in mental health / substance use services following the access intervention.

Finally, only six of the 24 unique studies reported patient-level outcomes. Of those, three reported no significant impact of access on outcomes. One study of PCMH integration found that integration led to better scores on a measure of physical functioning and a second found that a telemedicine intervention led to improvements on mental health related quality of life. A third found mixed results in terms of condition-specific patient-level outcomes.

LIMITATIONS

There were several important limitations to this study. First, we identified a number of well designed studies that examined access interventions, but they were not included in our review because they did not include data regarding either actual or perceived access outcomes. Therefore, there may be studies that were designed to assess the impact of interventions on access that are not included in this review. We suggest that future research examining access interventions collect and compare measures of perceived and actual access across groups. Further, given the small number of high quality studies and the relatively small number of studies in support of a specific intervention, all findings require further validation.

RECOMMENDATIONS FOR FUTURE RESEARCH

Key Questions #1 and #1a: Additional research is warranted to further define the relationship between variation in access and variation in system-level and patient-level outcomes. To date, most research has focused on the impact of straight-line distance on utilization but actual travel time and ease of transportation (measures of perceived access) and wait times (for appointments and in clinics) may be important factors to consider. Few studies of inpatient care have looked at associations with ability to pay for care or social support. Many of the studies used existing databases which allow for large sample sizes but limit analyses to variables captured in those databases. For example, few studies could examine the role of non-VA care. Finally, other elements of access (e.g., ways in which veterans needing care enter the VA health care system, costs of care) and other outcomes (e.g., patient satisfaction, improved health status) should be addressed.

Key Questions #2 and #2a: There is a burgeoning literature base which suggests that interventions to increase access to healthcare may be efficacious; however, additional research is required. During our literature review, we identified a number of well designed studies that examined access interventions, but they were not included in our review because they did not include either actual or perceived access outcomes.[58-62] When studying interventions hypothesized to improve access, measures of access need to be collected and compared across groups. Not only would this strengthen the evidence base, but would also provide data regarding new / different barriers that may emerge in the intervention condition (e.g., technical difficulties with telehealth services), and lessen the efficacy of the intervention.

The strength of evidence was strongest for the studies that examined the impact of copayments on access (medication adherence). Future research should examine whether a decrease in copayments would increase access to needed medications. Further, the cost of copayment decreases as a method of improving access should be compared to the cost of other, more resource intensive access interventions to determine the relative cost-effectiveness of decreasing medication copayments.

The interventions varied tremendously in their complexity and number of components. Moving forward, it will be important to determine the necessary and sufficient components of access interventions. Further, researchers must begin to focus on the relationship between the level of intervention complexity and the size of its impact on access and other outcomes. Shiner et al.,[38] who explored the effectiveness of five levels of PCMH integration, is an example of how such intensity-benefit analyses may be conducted. Within such studies, it will also be important to determine the cost of the intervention and the impact of the intervention on future healthcare costs (some included studies did report cost savings, but those outcomes were not extracted). Then, the complexity, intensity, and cost of the interventions can be considered when evaluating their impact on access. Such cost / benefit analyses may reveal significant benefits to using new, less resource intensive modes of accessing care (e.g., web-based, e-mail, text messaging). Further, moving forward, it will be important to determine the quality of care that veterans are receiving with increased access. As Shiner et al.[38] appropriately asked in their title "Access to What?", in addition to broad measures of access, future research should focus on access to evidence-based, quality care.

Finally, a majority of the articles focused on utilization and few examined patient-level outcomes. The data regarding utilization are difficult to interpret as it is unclear whether increased utilization is a desired, positive outcome. Further, given that utilization data were not linked to patient-level outcomes, it is not possible to determine whether the additional care was necessary and high quality. For example, one of the two good quality RCTs included in the review found that increased access to primary care actually resulted in higher rates of hospital readmission.[45] The question of whether more, higher intensity care results in better outcomes has previously been examined in the literature and the findings clearly suggest that access to more care / higher intensity care does not consistently lead to better outcomes, and at times, may be associated with poorer outcomes.[63-65] Given this, we recommend a decreased focus on utilization as an outcome and suggest that if utilization is included as an outcome, it is either specific to the type of care received (e.g., receipt of evidence-based care) or linked to patient-level outcomes. Finally, research on patient-level outcomes must be priority in the future. Such work will be challenging because there are a number of variables might impact both access and outcomes (e.g., comorbidities). Thus, rigorous, highly controlled research will be needed to ensure that increased access is resulting in improved health for veterans.

REFERENCES

1. Fortney J. "A re-conceptualization of access for 21ˢᵗ century healthcare." Oral presentation given to the VA Health Services Research & Development Service Timely Topics of Interest Cyber Seminar Series, August 2010.

2. Mayo-Smith MF. "Access issues within VA offer challenges, research opportunities." FORUM, VA Health Services Research & Development Service, July 2008.

3. Weeks WB. "Access to care: a VA research agenda." FORUM, VA Health Services Research & Development Service, July 2008.

4. Agency for Healthcare Research and Quality. 2007 National Healthcare Disparities Report. Rockville, MD: U.S. Department of Health and Human Services, Agency for Healthcare Research and Quality, AHRQ Pub. No. 08-0041, February 2008.

5. Demakis, JG. "Rural health-improving access to improve outcomes." Management Brief, Health Services Research & Development Service, No. 13:1-3, Jan 2000.

6. Institute of Medicine Committee on Monitoring Access to Personal Health Care Services. Access to health care in America. Millman M. (Ed.). Washington, CD: National Academy Press, 1993.

7. Miller LJ. "Improving access to care in the VA health system: A progress report." FORUM, VA Health Services Research & Development Service, June 2001.

8. Harris RP, Helfand M, Woolf SH, et al. (2001). Current methods of the U.S. Preventive Services Task Force: A review of the process. Am J Prev Med 2001;20(3S):21-35.

9. Fortney JC, Booth BM, Blow FC, Bunn JY, Loveland Cook CAl. The effects of travel barriers and age on the utilization of alcoholism treatment aftercare. Am J Drug Alcohol Abuse 1995;21:391-406.

10. Piette JD, Moos RH. The influence of distance on ambulatory care use, death, and readmission following a myocardial infarction. Health Serv Res 1996;31:573-91.

11. Prentice JC, Pizer SD. Delayed access to health care and mortality. Health Serv Res 2007;42:644-62.

12. Prentice JC, Pizer SD. Wait times and hospitalizations for ambulatory care sensitive conditions. Health Serv Outcomes Res Methods 2008;8:1-18.

13. Burgess JF Jr, DeFiore DA. The effect of distance to VA facilities on the choice and level of utilization of VA outpatient services. Soc Sci Med 1994;39:95-104.

14. Druss BG, Rosenheck RA. Use of medical services by veterans with mental disorders. Psychosomatics 1997;38:451-8.

15. Elhai JD, Grubaugh AL, Richardson JD, Egede LE, Creamer M. Outpatient medical and mental healthcare utilization models among military veterans: results from the 2001 National Survey of Veterans. J Psychiatr Res 2008;42:858-67.

16. Fasoli DR, Glickman ME, Eisen SV. Predisposing characteristics, enabling resources and need as predictors of utilization and clinical outcomes for veterans receiving mental health services. Med Care 2010;48;288-95.

17.   Fortney JC, Owen R, Clothier J. Impact of travel distance on the disposition of patients presenting for emergency psychiatric care. J Behav Health Serv Res 1999;26:104-8.

18.   Holloway JJ, Medendorp SV, Bromberg J. Risk factors for early readmission among veterans. Health Serv Res 1990;25:213-37.

19.   Hynes DM, Koelling K, Stroupe K, et al. Veterans' access to and use of Medicare and Veterans Affairs health care. Med Care 2007;45:214-23.

20.   LaVela SL, Smith B, Weaver FM, Miskevics SA. Geographical proximity and health care utilization in veterans with SCI&D in the USA. Soc Sci Med 2004;59:2387-99.

21.   McCarthy JF, Blow FC. Older patients with serious mental illness: sensitivity to distance barriers for outpatient care. Med Care 2004;42:1073-80.

22.   McCarthy JF, Blow FC, Valenstein M, et al. Veterans Affairs health system and mental health treatment retention among patients with serious mental illness: evaluating accessibility and availability barriers. Health Serv Res 2007;42:1042-60.

23.   Morgan RO, Petersen LA, Hasche JC, et al. VHA pharmacy use in veterans with Medicare drug coverage. Am J Manag Care 2009;15:e1-e8.

24.   Petersen LA, Byrne MM, Daw CN, Hasche J, Reis B, Pietz K. Relationship between clinical conditions and use of Veterans Affairs health care among Medicare-enrolled veterans. Health Serv Res 2010;45:762-791.

25.   Schmitt SK, Phibbs CS, Piette JD. The influence of distance on utilization of outpatient mental health aftercare following inpatient substance abuse treatment. Addict Behav 2003;28:1183-92.

26.   Cunningham WE, Hays RD, Williams KW, Beck KC, Dixon WJ, Shapiro MF. Access to medical care and health-related quality of life for low-income persons with symptomatic human immunodeficiency virus. Med Care 1995;33:739-54.

27.   Gamache GR, Rosenheck RA, Tessler R. Factors predicting choice of provider among homeless veterans with mental illness. Psychiatr Serv 2000;51:1024-8.

28.   Gordon AJ, Haas GL, Luther JF, Hilton MT, Goldstein G. Personal, medical, and healthcare utilization among homeless veterans served by metropolitan and nonmetropolitan veteran facilities. Psychol Serv 2010;7:65-74.

29.   Gurley D, Novins DK, Jones MC, Beals J, Shore JH, Manson SM. Comparative use of biomedical services and traditional healing options by American Indian veterans. Psychiatr Serv 2001;52:68-74.

30.   West A, Weeks WB. Physical and mental health and access to care among nonmetropolitan veterans health administration patients younger than 65 years. J Rural Health 2006;22:9-16.

31.   West AN, Weeks WB, Wallace AE. Rural veterans and access to high-quality care for high-risk surgeries. Health Serv Res 2008;43:1737-1751.

32.   Fortney JC, Borowsky SJ, Hedeen AN, Maciejewski ML, Chapko MK. VA Community-Based Outpatient Clinics: access and utilization performance measures. Med Care 2002;40:561-9.

33.   Fortney JC, Maciejewski ML, Warren JJ, Burgess JF Jr. Does improving geographic access to VA primary care services impact patients' patterns of utilization and costs? Inquiry 2005;42:29-42.

34.   Fortney JC, Steffick DE, Burgess JF Jr., Maciejewski ML, Petersen LA. Are primary care services a substitute or complement for specialty and inpatient services? Health Serv Res 2005;40:1422-42.

35.   Rosenheck R. Primary care satellite clinics and improved access to general and mental health services. Health Serv Res. 2000;35:777-90.

36.   Borowsky SJ, Nelson DB, Fortney JC, Hedeen AN, Bradley JL, Chapko MK. VA community-based outpatient clinics: performance measures based on patient perceptions of care. Med Care 2002;40:578-86.

37.   Morgester WA, Biggs CJ. Community-based VHA clinics: effect on patient satisfaction and re-source utilization. J Healthc Qual 2002;24:34-8.

38.   Shiner B, Watts BV, Pomerantz A, et al. Access to what? An evaluation of the key ingredients to effective advanced mental health access at a VA medical center and its affiliated community-based outreach clinics. Mil Med 2009;174:1024-32.

39.   Watts BV, Shiner B, Pomerantz A, Stender P, Weeks WB. Outcomes of a quality improvement project integrating mental health into primary care. Qual Saf Health Care 2007;16:378-81.

40.   Druss BG, Rohrbaugh RM, Levinson CM, Rosenheck RA. Integrated medical care for patients with serious psychiatric illness. Arch Gen Psychiatry 2001;58:861-8.

41.   Saxon AJ, Malte CA, Sloan Kl, et al. Randomized trial of onsite versus referral primary medical care for veterans in addictions treatment. Med Care 2006;44:334-42.

42.   Blue-Howells J, McGuire J, Nakashima J. Co-location of health care services for homeless veterans: A case study of innovation in program implementation. Soc Work Health Care 2008;47:219-231.

43.   McGuire J, Gelberg L, Blue-Howells J, Rosenheck RA. Access to primary care for homeless vet-erans with serious mental illness or substance abuse: a follow-up evaluation of co-located primary care and homeless social services. Admin Policy Ment Health 2009;36:255-64.

44.   Ritchie C, Weiland D, Tully C, Rose J, Sims R, Bodner E. Coordination and advocacy for rural elders (CARE): a model of rural case management with veterans. Gerontologist 2002;42:399-405.

45.   Weinberger M, Oddone EZ, Henderson WG. Does increased access to primary care reduce hospital readmissions? Veterans Affairs Cooperative Study Group on Primary Care and Hospital Readmission. New Engl J Med 1996;334:1441-7.

46.   Barnett TE, Chumbler NR, Vogel WB, Beyth RJ, Qin H, Kobb R. The effectiveness of a care co-ordination home telehealth program for veterans with diabetes mellitus: a 2- year follow-up. Am J Manag Care 2006;12:467-74.

47.   Hopp F, Woodbridge P, Subramanian U, Copeland L, Smith D, Lowery J. Outcomes associated with a home care telehealth intervention. Telemed J E Health 2006;12:297-307.

48.   Wakefield BJ, Buresh KA, Flanagan JR, Kienzle MG. Interactive video specialty consultations in long-term care. J Am Geriatr Soc 2004;52:789-93.

49.   Wilkins E, Lowery JC, Goldfarb S. Feasibility of virtual wound care. Adv Skin Wound Care 2007;20:275-8.

50.   McFall M, Malte C, Fontana A, Rosenheck RA. Effects of an outreach intervention on use of mental health services by veterans with posttraumatic stress disorder. Psychiatr Serv 2000;51:369-74.

51.   Maciejewski ML, Bryson CL, Perkins M, et al. Increasing copayments and adherence to diabetes, hypertension, and hyperlipidemic medications. Am J Manag Care 2010;15:e20-34.

52.   Zeber JE, Grazier KL, Valenstein M, Blow FC, Lantz PM. Effect of a medication copayment increase in veterans with schizophrenia. Am J Manag Care 2007;13:335-46.

53.   Doshi JA, Zhu J, Lee BY, Kimmel SE, Volpp KG. Impact of a prescription copayment increase on lipid-lowering medication adherence in veterans. Circulation 2009;119:390-7.

54.   Stroupe KT, Smith BM, Lee TA, et al. Effect of increased copayments on pharmacy use in the Department of Veterans affairs. Med Care 2007;45:1090-7.

55.   Hagedorn H, Dieperink E, Dignmann D, et al. Integrating hepatitis prevention services into a sub stance use disorder clinic. J Subst Abuse Treat 2007;32:391-8.

56.   Bates BE, Kurichi JE, Marshall CR, Reker D, Maislin G, Steineman MG. Does the presence of a specialized rehabilitation unit in a Veterans Affairs facility impact referral for rehabilitative care after a lower-extremity amputation? Arch Phys Med Rehabil 2007;88:1249-55.

57.   Rodriguez KL, Appelt CJ, Young AJ, Fox AR. African American veterans' experiences with mobile geriatric care. J Health Care Poor Underserved 2007;18:44-53.

58.   Tuerk PW, Yoder M, Ruggiero KJ, Gross DF, Acierno R. A pilot study of prolonged exposure therapy for posttraumatic stress disorder delivered via telehealth technology. J Trauma Stress 2010;23:116-23.

59.   Bauer MS, McBride L, Shea N, Gavin C, Holden F, Kendall S. Impact of an easy-access VA clinic-based program for patients with bipolar disorder. Psychiatr Serv 1997;48:491-6.

60.   Bauer MS, McBride L, Williford WO, et al. Collaborative care for bipolar disorder: Part II. Impact on clinical outcome, function, and costs. Psychiatr Serv 2006;57:937-45.

61.   Boutelle KN, Dubbert P, Vander Weg M. A pilot study evaluating a minimal contact telephone and mail weight management intervention for primary care patients. Eat Weight Disord 2005;10:e1-5.

62.   Egede LE, Frueh CB, Richardson LK, et al. Rationale and design: telepsychology service delivery for depressed elderly veterans. Trials [Electronic Resource] 2009;10:22.

63.   Fisher, ES. Avoiding the unintended consequences of growth in medical care. JAMA. 1999;281:446-53.

64.   Fisher, ES. Medical care — is more always better? N Engl J Med 2003;349:1665-7.

65.   Sirovich BE, Gottlieb, DJ, Welch HG, Fisher, ES. Regional variations in health care intensity and physician perceptions of quality of care. Ann Intern Med 2006;144:641-9.

APPENDIX A. SEARCH STRATEGY

Database: Ovid MEDLINE(R) <1950 to May Week 4 2010>

Search Strategy:

----

1 exp *Health Services Accessibility/ (34616)

2 limit 1 to (english language and humans and yr="1990 -Current" and "all adult (19 plus years)" and english) (6577)

3 *Veterans/ (4309)

4 *United States Department of Veterans Affairs/ (1252)

5 *Hospitals, Veterans/ (2008)

6 or/3-5 (6992)

7 2 and 6 (75)

8 access.mp. (114750)

9 6 and 8 (287)

10 limit 10 to (english language and humans and yr="1990 -Current" and "all adult (19 plus years)" and english) (182)

11 7 or 10 (209)

APPENDIX B. PEER REVIEW COMMENTS AND AUTHOR RESPONSES

REVIEWER COMMENT	RESPONSE
1. Are the objectives, scope, and methods for this review clearly described?	
Three specific comments about the search strategy:	
a. The primary (or only) barrier to access that appears to be addressed in KQ1 was distance. However, there are numerous other relevant barriers and facilitators to access that I expected to be addressed in KQ1, including price/income, social support, health literacy, and access to other health systems (e.g., Medicare). These are all implied by the Potential Moderators in Figure 1, but only distance receives attention. A Medline search limited to "Health Services Accessibility" in Appendix A missed articles that address these issues, and studies that I expected to be included in KQ2.	a. Thank you for the suggestion. We revised the KQ1 section to highlight other barriers and facilitators to access. To re-do the search at this point would markedly expand the scope and practice.
	b. The inclusion and exclusion criteria are outlined in the method section. We attempted to clarify that for KQ1, we included only studies that reported on how a measure of access impacted system-level or patient-level outcomes. Further, for KQ2, we included only studies that reported impact of the intervention on a measure of access (objective, subjective, or satisfaction with access).
b. It would be helpful to delineate whether specific types of studies were explicitly excluded or not considered for some reason. There may not have been such exclusion, but if so it should be mentioned.	c. We clarified that the types of interventions were not a priori categories used in the search, but rather, we developed after the search as a way to more cohesively present the findings. A brief description of each of the types of interventions is now presented in Table 2.
c. Clear definitions of the seven types of interventions discussed in KQ2 would be informative for the reader who had some other studies in mind and wondered what category they would fall in.	
2. Is there any indication of bias in our synthesis of the evidence?	
As mentioned in Comment #1 above, I expected to see a review of other barriers to access besides distance in response to KQ1. Not sure if it represents a bias per se.	As noted above, we revised the KQ1 section.
I expected there to be a number of studies reviewed in KQ2 that were not and it isn't clear to me why they weren't included. Not sure if it represents a bias per se.	Thank you for the suggested references. We have reviewed these citations and have included those that met our inclusion criteria.
a. In the section on CBOCs, I expected to see the following cites: Maciejewski et al. BMC HSR 2007, Liu et al. HSR 2010..	
b. In the section on intensive case management, I expected to see Bosworth Ann Intern Med 2009 and Am Heart J 2009; Piette 2001 (diabetes); Heisler Ann Intern Med 2010; other self-management trials by VA researchers	
c. The copay section should include papers by Stroupe Medical Care 2007 and Doshi Circulation 2009	
3. Are there any published or unpublished studies that we may have overlooked?	
a. For the section on page 6 (discussion of 2 Medicare papers), there are a number of papers (Wright, Petersen, Weeks, West, Liu, Morgan) that also address this issue of choice of VA or non-VA facilities that should be incorporated.	a. We have reviewed the suggested references and included those that met our inclusion criteria.
b. Given the SOTA focus on e-health applications to improve access, all published e-health interventions (MyHealtheVet, telemedicine, nurse case management via telephone or Web) should be reviewed and included.	b. We have included studies of e-health applications if they met our inclusion criteria and presented data regarding the impact of the intervention on a measure of access (objective, subjective, or satisfaction with access).

4. Additional comments

Comment	Response
This is a good paper on an important topic. It is even more important now that the VA has mandated 14 day access to all clinics. This mandate makes it even more important to carefully understand the literature and its limitations.	Thank you.
I strongly feel there needs to be much more attention to the quality of studies synthesized in this paper. I would like some summary for each section of the types and quality of the studies contributing data to the discussion. There seems to be little discrimination between RCTs and cross-sectional studies as an example --- no clear sense of guidance from the authors on how the reader should weight the study findings.	We agree and have added information about study type and quality.
I believe that "wait times" and "distance from the VA" should be considered separately – one is controlled by the VA and one is controlled by the patient. It seems to me that all of the studies evaluating patient health outcomes and their association with distance from the VA (or any other medical system) are almost meaningless. Unless the studies very carefully control for health status, SES, patient choices, etc., the findings are not useful, other than for the evaluation of access. It is impossible to know whether patients more distant from medical care are similar to those that are closer. Patients choose where they live for complex reasons some of which could be controlled for if assessed but some which might not ever be able to be accounted for in an observational study. If this body of literature includes studies that attempted to control for other factors, the authors need to describe this and weight the studies by their attempts to control for these potential confounders. On the other hand, waiting times are within the control of the VA and are much less likely to be confounded by patient factors. I feel strongly that each of these categories should be a subsection relating to key questions 1 and 1a. In addition to better descriptions/weighting of the studies, these issues should be more fully explored in the discussion.	Thank you for the suggestion. However, in light of the suggestion to include other barriers/facilitators, we modified the response to KQ1 to highlight factors other than distance and wait time. We organized the section by clinical area. We have rated the quality of the included studies and control of potential confounding factors was an important consideration in assigning the quality rating.
I consistently find putting the summary of findings at the beginning of a section awkward and confusing. The summary should come at the end, not the beginning of a section.	We moved the summary of findings to the end of each section.
The data on copayments seems fairly strong yet is not discussed much if at all in the discussion. This seems like fairly good and important data that could make a difference to patient care at the VA.	We agree and we added a discussion of the copayment studies to both the conclusions and future research sections.

For KQ1, I recommend describing the literature you found under each subsection. For example, it the "system-level outcomes" section, I think it would be much easier to follow the studies if you describe what you found for these types of studies there rather than in the literature summary paragraph on page 4 that precedes this section. I would like to know more about these 17 studies. Were they cross-sectional, prospective or retrospective cohort studies, or RCTs and what was their quality? I would like to know how many of each of these contribute to the section. It might even make sense to divide KQ1 into 2 parts rather than include both system level and patient level outcomes in one KQ. Few of the studies contribute to both outcomes.	Thank you for the suggestion. We have added information about study design and quality to the text.
I would like to see more epidemiologic thought in the discussion. The issue of more care equating to with improved care deserves a little more discussion than it was given. The Weinberger paper should be discussed more fully in this regard.	Thank you for the suggestion. We expanded our discussion of the issue as to whether more care equates with better care and reference Weinberger 1996 as an example.

APPENDIX C. EVIDENCE TABLES

Table 1. Studies examining variation in outcomes associated with variation in access (KQ1)

Author, Year Study Quality^	Study Design, Sample Size	Inclusion/Exclusion Criteria	Outcomes Assessed Covariates	Impact on System-Level Outcomes	Impact of Access on Patient-Level Outcomes	Interactions
Burgess & DeFiore, 1994[13] Fair	Cross-sectional n=6,386 veterans (national survey)	Inclusion: Responders to the 1987 Survey of Veterans (SOV)	Choice of VA over other outpatient options and amount of VA outpatient use Distance, characteristics of closest VA facility, age	1) Likelihood of using VA for outpatient services decreased as distance increased up to 60 miles (little change beyond 60 miles) 2) For veterans who choose some outpatient VA services, distance has a smaller additional effect on number of visits	N/A*	Effect of distance on number of outpatient VA visits is greatest for those >65 yrs
Cunningham et al., 1995[26] Fair	Cross-sectional n=205 HIV infected patients interviewed at one VA (n=28) and one county-run hospital (n=177)	Inclusion: ≥18 years of age, first seen with at least one of a) sustained fever, b) involuntary weight loss, c) sustained diarrhea Exclusion: cognitive impairment	Overall perceived access, temporal access, health related quality of life (HRQOL) Age, gender, race, mode of HIV transmission, education, income, marital status, log of CD4 counts, symptoms	Prevalence of access problems: Cost of care: 49% Office hours: 48% Location: 34% Appt. w/ Specialists: 15% Transportation time >30 min: 55% >1 hour: 17% # days to schedule urgent appt >1 day 50% >2 days 23% Office wait time >1 hour 54% >2 hours 32%	Better overall perceived access to care associated with better HRQOL for 8 of 11 scales including overall quality of life (p<0.001); temporal access scores not significantly associated with HRQOL	Adjusted access scores for VA care significantly (p<0.05) higher† for: a. covering cost of care (vs. uninsured) b. availability of emergency care (vs. uninsured or Medi-Cal) c. availability of hospital care (vs. uninsured) d. office wait time (vs. uninsured or Medi-Cal) VA scores significantly (p<0.05) lower for: a. convenience of contacting provider (vs. uninsured or Medi-Cal) b. transportation time (vs. Medi-Cal)
Druss & Rosenheck, 1997[14] Fair	Cohort n=44,533 veterans nationwide	Inclusion: discharged to the community from VA inpatient psychiatry and substance abuse programs during 6 month period in 1994-95, primary psychiatric or substance abuse disorder and secondary medical disorders	Four measures representing access, timeliness, and intensity of outpatient medical services utilization System-facility factors (e.g., region, hospital size, academic emphasis, specialization in mental health care) Predisposing factors (e.g., age, gender, race, marital status, diagnosis of psychiatric or substance abuse) Enabling factors (e.g., compensation, proximity, receipt of psychiatric or substance abuse services within 30 days of discharge) Illness leading to seeking treatment	Proximity to VA clinic, receipt of VA compensation payments, mental health follow-up within 30 days of discharge, and psychiatric diagnosis associated (p<0.01) with receipt of medical-surgical follow-up within 6 month post-discharge, receipt of medical services within 30 days post-discharge, number of days from discharge until first medical visit (among those with a visit), and number of visits in 6 month post-discharge	N/A	N/A

Interventions to Improve Veterans' Access to Care

Author, Year Study Quality^	Study Design, Sample Size	Inclusion/Exclusion Criteria	Outcomes Assessed Covariates	Impact on System-Level Outcomes	Impact of Access on Patient-Level Outcomes	Interactions
Elhai et al., 2008[15] Good	Cross-sectional n=20,048 veterans who completed 2001 National Survey of Veterans	Inclusion: non-institutionalized, identified by random digit dialing and from lists of patients enrolled in VA health care or receiving VA compensation or pensions	Treatment use over past 12 months – VA and non-VA outpatient health care visits, VA and non-VA mental health treatment Gender, age, race, education level, marital status, combat exposure; health insurance status, employment status, urban/rural residence; disability status, SF-12 mental and physical health components	Outpatient health care: 1) VA visit counts associated with younger age, unmarried status, lack of health insurance, unemployment, disability rating, poorer physical health (all p<0.01) 2) non-VA visits associated with female gender, older age, college education, unemployment, disability rating, poorer physical and mental health (all p<0.01) Mental healthcare use: 1) VA use associated with younger age, unmarried status, unemployment, lack of health insurance 2) non-VA use associated with female gender, younger age, college education, unmarried status, unemployed, urban residence, and poorer physical and mental health	N/A	N/A
Fasoli et al., 2010[16] Fair	Cohort n=421 veterans from 2 VA mental health centers in Boston area	Inclusion: English speaking, receiving inpatient or outpatient mental health service (MHS), mid 2004 to mid 2006	MHS utilization (outpatient, inpatient, residential), Global Assessment of Functioning (GAF), and Behavior and Symptoms Identification Scale-24 (BASIS-24) after 3 months Demographics, partial self-pay for care, employment, social support, emotional support, problems getting to treatment, housing, level of care at enrollment, baseline GAF and BASIS-24, diagnoses, comorbidities, disability, service connection, MHS use 6 months prior	1) Increased outpatient utilization among patients who reported fewer access problems and no social support (both p<0.05); greatest predictor of use was clinical need 2) Increased inpatient hospitalization associated with homelessness; greatest predictor was clinical need	GAF and BASIS-24 at 3 months not significantly related to access or outpatient utilization; inpatient hospitalization predicted worse GAF and BASIS-24 at 3 months	N/A

Author, Year Study Quality^	Study Design, Sample Size	Inclusion/Exclusion Criteria	Outcomes Assessed Covariates	Impact on System-Level Outcomes	Impact of Access on Patient-Level Outcomes	Interactions
Fortney et al., 1995[9] Good	Cohort n=4,631 male veterans from 33 VA treatment programs	Inclusion: Primary diagnosis of alcohol dependence; completed VA inpatient program, discharged with outpatient appointment, resided in primary service area of the inpatient facility	Attendance at aftercare appointment within 30 days of discharge Travel distance, socio-medical characteristics (age, race, severity of illness, marital status, level of urbanization)	Patients living farther from the treatment program were less likely to choose to attend their aftercare appointment as were urban residing (with distance held constant) patients and unmarried patients	N/A	Older patients and rural residents more negatively affected by distance than younger patients or urban residents
Fortney et al., 1999[17] Fair	Cross-sectional n=109 veterans from Little Rock, AR VAMC	Inclusion: Walk-ins to Psychiatric Evaluation Clinic in Emergency Medicine Service Exclusion: missing data, out of state residence, restricted medical records	Disposition (admission or outpatient appointment) Age, marital status, employment status, ethnicity, travel distance, number of psychiatric and medical comorbidities, number of psychosocial and environmental problems, current GAF	Admissions: 17% of those living <60 mi from VAMC; 43% of those living 60+ mi from VAMC (p=0.003); controlling for case mix OR=4.8 [1.06-22.1]; age >65 and lower GAF also associated with increased likelihood of admission	N/A	N/A
Gamache et al., 2000[27] Poor	Cross-sectional n= 663 homeless veterans in Access to Community Care and Effective Services & Supports program in 9 states	Inclusion: homeless, serious mental illness, not involved in ongoing community treatment	Lifetime use of VA health services Age, gender, marital status, race/ethnicity, education, military service era, addiction severity, health problems, service connection, income, residence in city with VA hospital	Veterans with service connected disabilities or non-service connected pensions or veterans living in cities with VA medical centers or hospitals were more likely to have used VA services (all p<0.05)	N/A	N/A
Gordon et al., 2010[28] Poor	Cross-sectional n=3,595 veterans interviewed FY† 2002-2003, VISN4	Inclusion: presently or recently homeless military veterans; identified in community, VA hospitals and clinics, veteran's centers, prisons	Use of any VA services in past 6 months Metropolitan/non-metropolitan location, demographics, military history, living situation, employment, medical history	Greater use associated with metropolitan location and VA financial support (p<0.001)	N/A	Significant interactions - metro/non-metro & use of services (p<0.05); Age, military service period, monthly income, time homeless, past alcohol or drug dependency

33

Author, Year / Study Quality^	Study Design, Sample Size	Inclusion/Exclusion Criteria	Outcomes Assessed / Covariates	Impact on System-Level Outcomes	Impact of Access on Patient-Level Outcomes	Interactions
Gurley et al., 2001[29] / Fair	Cross-sectional / n=621 male veterans from American Indian reservation communities in Southwest (n=316) and Northern Plains (n=305)	Inclusion: Vietnam service, living on or within 50 miles of reservation, born between 1930 and 1958 NOTE: VA services described by authors as more readily available for Northern Plains veterans	Use of VA, Indian Health, other biomedical health services, and traditional healer (inpatient in past year, outpatient in past 6 months)	Significantly greater (p≤ 0.05) use of VA services by veterans from Northern Plains reservation communities for physical and mental health problems; significantly greater (p≤ 0.001) use of traditional healer by Southwest reservation veterans	N/A	N/A
Holloway et al., 1990[18] / Good	Cross-sectional / n=6,317 veterans with index admission to Ann Arbor VA Medical Center (data from random sample of 3,159 used to develop model)	Inclusion: discharged from internal medicine, surgery, intermediate care, or neurology services or a tertiary care VA medical center 1/1/81 to 12/31/82 Exclusion: patients admitted to psychiatry service, uncertainty about readmission	Early readmission (within 30 days of discharge) for any reason Location of residence (relative to VA medical center), number of surgical procedures, compensation and pension status, readmission risk class (based on diagnosis-related group), bed section of discharge, age	Increased distance of county of residence from VAMC associated with non-significant increased probability of early readmission; significantly increased probability if two or more surgeries performed, readmission risk above "very low," or patient on intermediate, neurology, or surgery service at discharge	N/A	N/A
Hynes et al., 2007[19] / Good	Cross-sectional / n=1,474,417 veterans in outpatient analysis n=416,455 veterans in inpatient analysis	Inclusion: veterans eligible to use VA and Medicare health care in 1999, had used VA health services between 1997 and 1999 Exclusion: veteran status unknown, missing or invalid zip code, lived in Puerto Rico or other US territory, ≤65 years old on 1/1/99, end-stage renal disease, enrolled in Medicare+Choice care	VA and Medicare use (outpatient and inpatient services) Age; gender; race; vital status; VISN; priority level in VA;, health status risk score; distance to nearest VA inpatient hospital, VA outpatient center, and Medicare inpatient hospital; ZIP code (for poverty level); number of physicians, general hospitals, and beds in county of residence	Outpatient: decreased likelihood of exclusive use of VA as distance to VA increased; older age, higher health risk status, urban residence, and more hospital beds in county also associated with decreased exclusive use of VA; black race, high VA priority level, and high poverty level associated with increased exclusive use of VA Inpatient services: same pattern (all p<0.01)	N/A	N/A

Author, Year Study Quality^	Study Design, Sample Size	Inclusion/Exclusion Criteria	Outcomes Assessed Covariates	Impact on System-Level Outcomes	Impact of Access on Patient-Level Outcomes	Interactions
LaVela et al., 2004[20] Fair	Cross-sectional n=8,983 veterans with spinal cord injuries and disorders	Inclusion: traumatic lesions or demyelinating disease of the spinal cord; intraspinal, nonmalignant neoplasms, vascular insults, cauda equina syndrome, inflammatory disease of the spine, unstable traumatic lesions of the spinal column Exclusion: multiple sclerosis; missing, invalid, or non U.S./ Puerto Rico zip code; mobile clinic use; VA residential care patient; home care and telehealth related clinic stops, no VA utilization	Number of outpatient visits; number of inpatient discharges History of illness, travel distance to actual facility used; travel distance to nearest facility, age, race, gender, marital status, level of injury	Patients utilized outpatient services less frequently when VA facilities were farther away from their residences (p<0.000); increased age, non-white race, and history of respiratory, kidney/urinary tract, circulatory, or digestive system disease associated with increased outpatient utilization (all p<0.01) Patients had less inpatient utilization if they lived at greater distances (p<0.000); history of illnesses of respiratory, skin/ subcutaneous tissue/breast, kidney/urinary tract, circulatory, or digestive systems associated with increased inpatient utilization (all p<0.02)	N/A	N/A
McCarthy & Blow, 2004[21] Fair	Cohort n=142,055 veterans from national VA registry	Inclusion: diagnosis of bipolar disorder, schizophrenia, or other psychosis in year FY 2000 with some VA contact in FY 1999 Exclusion: little or no willingness to seek VA care, homeless, stay of 150+ days, died in FY 2000	Total outpatient non-psychiatric visit days, total outpatient psychiatric visit days Age, gender, race/ethnicity, marital status, urban/rural residence, distance to nearest relevant VA provider; psychiatric diagnosis type; comorbidity level, initial treatment location of FY	Patients further from outpatient care had fewer outpatient non-psychiatric visit days; older age, married, female, rural residence, initial visit at outpatient non-psychiatric facility, and higher comorbidity rating associated with increased visit days (all p<0.01) Patients further from psychiatric services had fewer outpatient psychiatric visit days; initial visit at non-psychiatric facility, higher comorbidity rating, and rural residence also associated with fewer psychiatric visits (all p<0.001)	N/A	Negative effects of distance on outpatient non-psychiatric visits - greater for patients with schizophrenia than bipolar disorders and for patients >65 yrs; on outpatient psychiatric visits - greater for patients with schizophrenia and for ages 45 to 65 yrs.

Author, Year Study Quality^	Study Design, Sample Size	Inclusion/Exclusion Criteria	Outcomes Assessed Covariates	Impact on System-Level Outcomes	Impact of Access on Patient-Level Outcomes	Interactions
McCarthy et al., 2007[22] Fair	Cohort n=156,631 veterans nationwide	Inclusion: diagnosis of schizophrenia or bipolar disorder in FY 1998 Exclusion: missing data or Alaska resident	Time to first 12-month gap in 1) VA health services utilization and 2) VA mental health services (through the end of FY 2002) Age, gender, marital status, race/ethnicity, VA service connection status, homelessness, primary psychiatric diagnosis, comorbidity index, distance to nearest VA service site or VA provider of substantial psychiatric services, inpatient care in FY 1998, VA and non-VA inpatient beds per 1000 county residents	Risk of gap in health service utilization increased with increased distance to nearest VA facility, homelessness, inpatient stay in FY98, and unknown or non-white race; decreased with more VA beds; increased age, female gender, married, VA service connection, higher comorbidity score, diagnosis of schizophrenia (all p<0.05) Risk of gap in mental health utilization increased with residence further from VA psychiatric service site, age, female gender, non-white race, homelessness, higher comorbidity score, inpatient stay in FY98; decreased with married, VA service connection, diagnosis of schizophrenia (all p<0.05)	N/A	N/A
Morgan et al., 2009[23] Fair	Cross-sectional n=3,424,699 veterans	Inclusion: enrolled in VHA and Medicare for at least 1 month in 2002	VHA pharmacy use Health status, income, race/ethnicity, age, metropolitan/non-metropolitan status, participation in Medicaid, VA priority status	Decreased likelihood of using VHA pharmacy if enrolled in Medicare HMO plan with pharmacy benefits, older than 65 yrs, income of $20,000 or greater, female, priority status other than 1 (no copayment), Medicare state buy-in, resident of metropolitan statistical area, and patient at a teaching hospital Increased likelihood if Hispanic race and poorer health status	N/A	N/A
Petersen et al., 2010[24] Good	Cross-sectional n=1,943,129 veterans	Inclusion: inpatient or outpatient VA or Fee basis use FY 2003 & 2004 who were also Medicare enrollees (including < 65 yrs) Exclusion: missing priority classification, diagnostic data, or ZIP code; died in FY 2003 or 2004; ZIP code outside of US	Reliance on VA health care (overall, inpatient, outpatient) Age, gender, race, differential distance (distance to VA Medical Center minus distance to non-VA hospital), priority classification, aggregated conditions categories (ACCs)	Overall increased reliance on VA care if differential distance is lower, if under age 65, or if disability or low income VA priority classification; mental health and substance abuse ACCs significantly associated with increased reliance on VA care Similar results for outpatient care Patients with transplant and amputation ACCs more likely to have inpatient VA care; other ACCs associated with inpatient VA care included infectious and parasitic disorders, substance abuse, mental health disorders, and eye disorders	N/A	Interaction of age and distance was significant but parameter effects were less than main effects Mental health and diseases of eyes, ears, nose, and throat associated with increased reliance on VA care for <65 yr group Mental health, substance abuse, diabetes, and infectious diseases associated with increased VA care for ≥65 yr group

Author, Year Study Quality^	Study Design, Sample Size	Inclusion/Exclusion Criteria	Outcomes Assessed Covariates	Impact on System-Level Outcomes	Impact of Access on Patient-Level Outcomes	Interactions
Piette & Moos, 1996[10] Good	Cohort n=4,637 male veterans from national VA databases	Inclusion: Admitted to VA acute care hospital, discharge diagnosis of myocardial infarction (MI) Exclusion: Death or readmission within 90 days of index discharge; index length of stay >100 days, reside >100 mi from a source of VA care or >200 mi from admitting facility	Outcomes Assessed: Outpatient medical care visits within 30 and 90 days of discharge following acute MI admission; death from all causes or recurrent cardiac admission 91 to 365 days after discharge Covariates: Age, VA service connection, comorbidity index, alcoholism, teaching hospital, catheterization or revascularization procedure	Patients with service connected disability, over age 55, with comorbid conditions, discharged from a teaching hospital, and having revascularization are more likely to have 1 or more visits within 30 days; patients with history of alcohol abuse and living more than 20 miles from admitting hospital were less likely (all p<0.05); similar pattern for 1 or more visits within 90 days except comorbidity, alcoholism, and hospital type not related	Age greater than 55, comorbidities, and distance greater than 20 miles associated with increased risk of death within 1 year; revascularization procedure and any VA ambulatory care in 90 days after index visit associated with decreased risk of death (all p<0.05); age greater than 65, comorbidities, and any VA ambulatory care in 90 days associated with increased risk of readmission (all p<0.05)	N/A
Prentice & Pizer, 2007[11] Good	Cohort n=37,489 veterans from 89 VAMCs	Inclusion: veterans ≥65 years old who visited at least one of three types of VA geriatric outpatient clinics between 10/1/00 and 6/30/01 and survived through 9/30/01	Outcomes Assessed: 6-month mortality (odds of dying between 10/1/01 and 3/31/02) Covariates: Age, gender, principal diagnoses, comorbidity index, preventable hospitalization in past year, service connected disability (50% or greater); facility 3-month mortality rate, facility wait time	N/A	Facility-level wait times of ≥31 days associated with significantly higher mortality; increased age, ≥ 50% service connected disability, preventable hospitalization, higher comorbidity index, and diagnosis of cancer or endocrine, neurological, psychiatric, pulmonary, or other disease associated with increased mortality; female gender associated with decreased mortality (all p<0.05)	N/A

Interventions to Improve Veterans' Access to Care

Author, Year Study Quality[A]	Study Design, Sample Size	Inclusion/Exclusion Criteria	Outcomes Assessed Covariates	Impact on System-Level Outcomes	Impact of Access on Patient-Level Outcomes	Interactions
Prentice & Pizer, 2008[12] Fair	Cohort n=33,431 veterans from 86 VAMCs	Inclusion: same as above except visits between 10/1/00 and 3/31/01, surviving through 6/30/01	Dependent variable: probability of hospitalization for an ambulatory care sensitive condition between 7/1/01 and 12/31/01 Age, gender, principal diagnoses, comorbidity index, ambulatory care sensitive condition (ACSC) hospitalization in past year; facility 3-month ACSC hospitalization rate	Facility-level wait times of ≥29 days associated with greater probability of hospitalization for ACSC compared to wait times of <22.5 days Facility average ACSC hospitalization rate, age, previous ACSC hospitalization, comorbidity index, and diagnosis of cancer, or endocrine, heart, or pulmonary disease also associated with increased probability of ACSC hospitalization (all p<0.02)	N/A	N/A
Schmitt et al., 2003[25] Fair	Cohort n=33,952 veterans from national VA databases	Inclusion: Admitted to substance abuse units, *eligible for outpatient aftercare* Exclusion: Discharged against medical advice, death or re-hospitalization within 90 days of index discharge, no valid zip code of residence	Use of any outpatient aftercare, number of mental health clinic visits within 90 days (for those with at least one visit) Comorbidity index	Increased likelihood of receiving aftercare if distance < 50 miles with greatest likelihood if distance <10 miles; age, married, service-connected eligibility, psychiatric comorbidity, substance use disorder, and teaching hospital associated with increased likelihood; medical comorbidity index 1, 2, or > 4 associated with decreased likelihood (all p<0.05) Volume of aftercare only greater if distance <10 miles (relative to >50 miles)	N/A	N/A
West & Weeks, 2006[30] Fair	Cross-sectional n=47,185 men who responded to the 2000 Behavioral Risk Factors Surveillance System telephone survey	Inclusion: Non-veteran or no longer in military service Exclusion: refused to say or didn't know whether ever in military service	Health in general, maximum poor health days (physical, mental, or limited usual activity in prior month), inability to afford needed care in past year	Non-metropolitan VA patients age 18 to 44 were significantly more likely to say they needed to see a doctor but could not because of cost than others of same age (p<0.005); among 45 to 64 year olds, VA patients (regardless of residence) more likely to report cost as a factor in accessing needed treatment	Self-reported health poorest for non-metropolitan veterans in VA care age 45 or older Days in past 30 of poor health highest for veterans in VA care regardless of residence (NOTE: veterans in VA care identified based on self-reported use of VA in past 12 months)	N/A

38

Author, Year Study Quality^	Study Design, Sample Size	Inclusion/Exclusion Criteria	Outcomes Assessed Covariates	Impact on System-Level Outcomes	Impact of Access on Patient-Level Outcomes	Interactions
West et al., 2008[31] Fair	Cross-sectional n=2,827,602 admissions (veterans hospitalized 2000 or 2001)	Inclusion: ≥65 yrs on date of admission, VA enrollee for whom Medicare claims were submitted; received any of 14 high-risk elective procedures	Utilization of VA or non-VA care, utilization of lower or higher quality care	Overall, 89% of heart surgeries, 84% of vascular surgeries, and 79% of cancer resections obtained in non-VA hospitals with little difference based on residence Urban residents more likely to obtain heart surgery (significant only for bypass grafting) and cancer resection in high performance hospitals; rural residents more likely to get vascular surgery in high performance hospitals Travel time to high performing hospital indicated that urban veterans had least travel burden; travel time to high performance hospital for heart surgery was shorter than to low performance, regardless of residence; no difference for vascular surgery	N/A	N/A

^Quality based on assessment of participant selection, outcomes assessment, and analysis (see text); †Access scores: 0=worst possible access, 100=best possible access; *N/A=Not available; †FY=fiscal year (October 1 to September 30 of the following year); NS=non-significant; VISN=Veterans Integrated Service Network

Table 2. Studies examining the efficacy of interventions designed to increase access for veterans (KQ2)

Community Based Outpatient Clinics (CBOCs) – Opening of satellite primary care clinics

Author, Title	Study Design, Study Quality	Setting	Patient Characteristics	Intervention / Comparator	Impact of Intervention on Access	Impact of Intervention on System-Level Outcomes	Impact on Intervention on Patient-Level Outcomes
Borowsky et al., 2002[36]	Cross-sectional survey, fair	44 CBOCS and 36 corresponding parent VAMCs	Randomly selected subset of veterans who had care at one of the selected CBOCs or VAMCs in the preceding six months.	Utilization of CBOCS / VAMC users	Veterans using CBOCs reported better access / timeliness and were more likely to report waits less than 20 minutes.	Veterans using CBOCS had more ratings of good / excellent visits; fewer problems in a variety of areas (e.g., emotional support, preferences, care coordination, education, courtesy).	N/A
Fortney et al., 2002[32]	Retrospective cohort analysis, fair	38 CBOCs and 32 parent VAMCs	All primary care patients treated at participating CBOCs or VAMCs.	Utilization of CBOCS / VAMC users	CBOC patients more likely to be new VA users.	CBOC patients had more primary care encounters and fewer specialty care encounters.	N/A
Fortney et al., 2005a[33], 2005b[34]	Quasi-experimental, fair	Fifteen CBOCS that offered primary care and opened during a six month period in 1997	All veterans living in the CBOC catchment area who had any VA service use in the six months before the CBOC opened. Included a matched group of veterans residing outside the catchment area of any new CBOCs	Implementation of CBOCs / pre-CBOC implementation	Decrease in travel distance to the closest VA facility for those in CBOC catchment area.	Decrease in travel distance predicted increase in primary care encounters; across diagnoses, those in CBOC catchment had more primary care visits, ancillary visits, and extended care physical health visits.	N/A
Morgester et al., 2002[37]	Case series, poor	One CBOC and the parent VAMC	Veterans with an appointment at the CBOC or VAMC during the recruitment period; veterans who lived in the CBOC catchment area and received non-VHA primary care	Utilization of CBOCS / utilization of VAMC or non-VA care	All three groups (VAMC, CBOC, non-VA care) reported few problems finding clinic (93-100%) and found the hours of operation convenient (97-100%). There were no statistical comparisons.	All three groups (VAMC, CBOC, non-VA care) reported satisfaction with care (93-100%); 82-83% of the VAMC and 90-93% of the CBOC veterans reported they had enough information about their condition and medication; 93% of CBOC and 90% of VAMC veterans felt they could care for themselves until next visit. There were no statistical comparisons.	N/A

Author, Title	Study Design, Study Quality	Setting	Patient Characteristics	Intervention / Comparator	Impact of Intervention on Access	Impact of Intervention on System-Level Outcomes	Impact on Intervention on Patient-Level Outcomes
Rosenheck et al., 2000[35]	Cohort Study, poor	All counties and the District of Columbia (compared those with and without CBOCS that opened from 1995-1998).	All veterans, based on census data	Implementation of CBOCs/ pre-CBOC implementation	Significantly greater proportion of veterans in counties with CBOCs accessed general VA medical services. In counties with CBOCs that had specialty mental health, mental health access greater.	N/A	N/A
Primary Care Mental Health Integration – Co-location of primary care and mental health services							
Blue-Howells et al., 2008[42]; McGuire et al., 2009[43]	Quasi-experimental, poor	Greater Los Angeles VA Medical Center	All veterans newly entering the Homeless Program	Implementation of integrated mental health, primary care, and homeless social services clinic / pre-implementation	Shorter wait time for initial primary care visit.	Improved preventive care, more primary care visits, lower emergency care service use.	No significant differences.
Druss et al., 2001[40]	RCT, fair	Large VA Medical Center	Veterans within mental health clinic without a primary care provider.	Integrated primary care services into mental health clinic / usual care.	Better self-reported access.	More primary care visits, fewer ER visits, improved preventive care, higher satisfaction	Higher (better) scores on the SF-36 physical component summary.
Saxon et al., 2006[41]	RCT, good	VA Puget Sound Health Care System	Veterans presenting for substance use treatment who did not have a primary care provider and had at least one chronic health or asymptomatic condition (e.g., high blood pressure).	Implemented an onsite (within the substance use clinic) primary care clinic / usual care	Shorter wait for initial primary care visit; greater odds of attending rescheduled initial visit; more likely to attend at least 1 primary care visit.	More likely to attend return primary care visits and averaged more primary care visits; less non-VA primary care. More likely to remain engaged in substance use treatment at 60 days.	No significant differences

Interventions to Improve Veterans' Access to Care

Author, Title	Study Design, Study Quality	Setting	Patient Characteristics	Intervention / Comparator	Impact of Intervention on Access	Impact of Intervention on System-Level Outcomes	Impact on Intervention on Patient-Level Outcomes
Shiner et al., 2009[38]	Cohort study, poor	Large VAMC and three CBOCs	Veterans who screened positive for depression in primary care.	Varying models of Primary Care Mental Health (PCMH). The VAMC had co-location of, and advance or open access to mental health providers; and standardized assessments. CBOC-A had walk in access one day per week, evaluation by a psychotherapist and a psychopharmacologically oriented provider, and standardized assessment. CBOC-B had a psychotherapist as part of the primary care team and back-up telepsychiatry services (by appointment). CBOC-C did not have PCMH, but mental health care was available at the CBOC. CBOC-D did not have PCMH and there was no mental health care on site (comparator).	Following implementation, VAMC and CBOC-A had increases in veterans seen in mental health within both 4 days and 30 days. CBOC-B had an increase of veterans seen within 30 days and percentage receiving optimal care. No differences in CBOCs C & D.	More patients at VAMC, CBOC-A, and CBOC-B received "optimal depression treatment."	N/A
Watts et al., 2007[39]	Cohort study, fair	White River Junction VAMC & CBOCs	Veterans who screened positive for depression in primary care	PCMH Integration / no PCMH integration	More patients received mental health services in primary care and were seen in mental health; shorter wait time for initial mental health appointment (all outcomes only significant for VAMC, not CBOCs)	More patients received "optimal depression treatment" (at VAMC, not CBOC)	N/A
Intensive Case Management – High intensity treatment coordination to facilitate identification of and access to needed services							
Ritchie et al., 2002[44]	Case series, poor	Two VAMCs	Elderly veterans in rural counties who were frail and at risk of repeated hospitalization	Pilot implementation of the Coordination and Advocacy for Rural Elders (CARE) program, which performs standardized, scheduled assessments; identifies problems; develops care plans; and tracks resolution of problems / no comparison	Over 56% received a medical service of referral / linkage.	N/A	N/A

Author, Title	Study Design, Study Quality	Setting	Patient Characteristics	Intervention / Comparator	Impact of Intervention on Access	Impact of Intervention on System-Level Outcomes	Impact on Intervention on Patient-Level Outcomes
Weinberger et al., 1996[45]	RCT, good	Nine VAMCs with diversity in location and academic affiliation	Hospitalized veterans with one of three chronic diseases without continuous primary care.	Implemented intensive primary care program designed to increase access to primary care; intervention included both an inpatient (e.g., follow-up planning, scheduling) and outpatient (e.g., appointment reminders, check-in phone call) components / usual care	Median time from hospital discharge to primary care shorter. Better satisfaction with self-reported access.	More likely to have at least one general medical clinic visit; more general medical clinic visits during six-months post-discharge; higher monthly hospital readmission rate; more days of hospital readmission; greater satisfaction with care.	No significant differences.
Telemedicine – Conducting encounters via telephone or interactive video conferencing							
Barnett et al., 2006[46]	Retrospective matched cohort analysis, fair	Four VAMCS in Florida, Puerto Rico, and Georgia	Older veterans with type two diabetes at high risk for multiple VA inpatient and outpatient visits.	Nurse coordinators monitored data from a home telehealth messaging device and made phone calls or scheduled appointments with the physician as necessary / treatment as usual	Care coordinator-initiated primary care clinic visits increased by 8.9%.	Decrease in all cause hospitalization, diabetes related hospitalizations (no longer significant after controlling for baseline A1C).	N/A
Hopp et al., 2006[47]	RCT, fair	Home care service line at a large VAMC in Indianapolis	All patients receiving home care services at the VAMC	In addition to traditional home care services, participants contacted VAMC using telehealth units / home care as usual	Most reported that their level of contact with VA providers increased.	No significant differences.	Improvement on the mental component summary of the Health Related Quality of Life scale
Wakefield et al., 2004[48]	Cross-sectional survey, poor	Two VAMCs and a long term care facility	Residents living at the Iowa Veterans Home.	Implemented interactive video conferencing to provide specialty consultation to veterans living at the long term care facility / no comparator	92% of veterans reported that using telemedicine made it easier to see the specialist.	81% of veterans reported satisfaction with the telemedicine consultation process.	N/A
Wilkins et al., 2007[49]	Pilot case series, poor	Two VAMCs without multidisciplinary wound care teams	Veterans with a wound who sought care at a VAMC without a wound care team.	Implemented telemedicine to seek consultations from a remote wound care team/ no comparator	Veterans reported that telemedicine was more convenient than travelling to wound care team.	Almost all (92.8%) participants were satisfied with telemedicine.	N/A

Author, Title	Study Design, Study Quality	Setting	Patient Characteristics	Intervention / Comparator	Impact of Intervention on Access	Impact of Intervention on System-Level Outcomes	Impact on Intervention on Patient-Level Outcomes
Outreach – Providing information about how to access care							
McFall et al., 2000[50]	RCT, poor	Large urban VAMC	Vietnam veterans living in vicinity of VAMC who are service-connected for PTSD without use of VA mental health or substance use services in the prior 12 months.	Outreach intervention with (1) a mailing which included information regarding PTSD treatment services and a letter from the PTSD program outlining three ways to initiate care (return postcard, call, or walk-in clinic), and (2) direct phone call during which veterans could ask about services, schedule an appointment, or address barriers / no intervention control group.	Significantly more likely to schedule an intake, present for intake session.	Significantly more likely to attend at least one follow-up session.	N/A
Copayments – Change in medication copayments							
Doshi et al., 2009[53]	Cohort study, fair	One large VAMC	Veterans on lipid-lowering medications	Increase in medication copayments from $2 to $7 / copayment exempt.	Lipid refill rates decreased for all veterans after copayment increase, but the decrease was small among those without copayment.	N/A	N/A
Maciejewski et al., 2010[51]	Cohort study, fair	Four large VAMCs	Veterans with diabetic or hypertension who had a prescription for those conditions (a portion of whom had copayments).	Increase in medication copayments from $2 to $7 / copayment exempt.	At the end of the study, lower adherence to diabetic and hypertensive medications among veterans with a copayment.	N/A	N/A
Stroupe et al., 2007[54]	Cohort study, fair	VA-Wide	A random sample of 5% of VA pharmacy users.	Increase in medication copayments from $2 to $7 / copayment exempt.	Those with a copayment received 8% fewer 30-day refills than those without payments.	N/A	N/A

Author, Title	Study Design, Study Quality	Setting	Patient Characteristics	Intervention / Comparator	Impact of Intervention on Access	Impact of Intervention on System-Level Outcomes	Impact on Intervention on Patient-Level Outcomes
Zeber et al., 2007[52]	Cohort study, fair	VA-wide	All veterans receiving a diagnosis of schizophrenia or schizoaffective disorder from 1998-1999 (a portion of whom had copayments).	Increase in medication copayments from $2 to $7 / copayment exempt.	For all medication and medical prescriptions: those exempt from copayments, prescriptions increased steadily throughout study, while for those with a copayment, growth slowed after price increase. For psychiatric drugs: for those exempt from copayments, prescriptions increased throughout study, while for those with a copay, use decreased after price increase.	Copayment group more likely to have psychiatric admission.	N/A
Other Access Interventions							
Bates et al., 2007[56]	Retrospective cohort analysis, poor	Two types of VAMCs, those with and without specialized rehab units	Veterans with lower-extremity amputations during study time frame.	Presence of Specialized Rehabilitation Unit (SRU) within the hospital / hospital without an SRU	No difference in the probability of receiving an initial rehabilitation consult; those in SRU more likely to receive specialized rehabilitation.	Longer length of non-ICU stays in SRU VAMCs.	Problems in peripheral circulation more common in non-SRU VAMCs, skin breakdown more common in SRU VAMCs.
Hagedorn et al., 2007[55]	Quasi-experimental, poor	A substance use clinic within a large VAMC	Veterans receiving services within the substance use clinic	Implementation of the Healthy Liver Program, designed to increase access to services for the prevention (vaccination), identification (testing), and treatment (referrals) of viral hepatitis within a substance use clinic / pre-implementation.	Testing for hepatitis increased, 94% of appropriate veterans started the vaccine series (vaccine was not available prior to implementation).	78% of those who learned they had hepatitis attended their intake at the hepatitis clinic.	N/A

Interventions to Improve Veterans' Access to Care

Author, Title	Study Design, Study Quality	Setting	Patient Characteristics	Intervention / Comparator	Impact of Intervention on Access	Impact of Intervention on System-Level Outcomes	Impact on Intervention on Patient-Level Outcomes
Rodriguez et al., 2007[57]	Qualitative study following implementation, poor	Two low income urban neigh-borhoods within the VA Pittsburgh Healthcare System	Elderly, urban, predominately African American men receiving care at one of the mobile care units.	Implemented a mobile care program, which had healthcare staff and resources to conduct basic medical care within the van/ no comparator.	Accessibility of care was mentioned 26 times in 18 interviews (2nd most common topic behind quality of care).	Quality of care was mentioned 28 times in 18 interviews.	N/A

www.ingramcontent.com/pod-product-compliance
Lightning Source LLC
Chambersburg PA
CBHW081622170526
45166CB00009B/3075